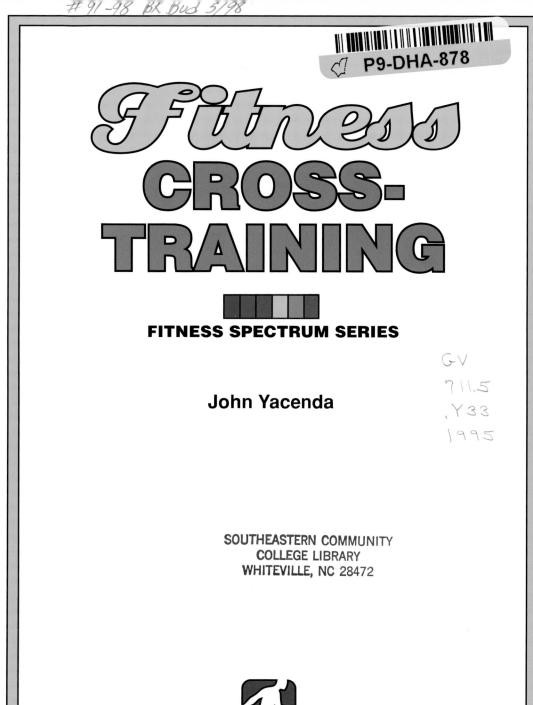

Fitness CROSS-TRAINING

FITNESS SPECTRUM SERIES

John Yacenda

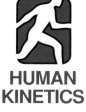

HUMAN KINETICS

For Benita, my wife, Tayesa, my daughter, Aida and Italo, the teenage children, and for all those who keep their commitments to themselves, and to those they love.

Library of Congress Catalog Information

Yacenda, John, 1947-
    Fitness cross-training / by John Yacenda.
       p.   cm. -- (Fitness spectrum series)
    Includes index.
    ISBN 0-87322-770-0
    1. Physical education and training.   2. Physical fitness.
    3. Exercise. I. Title. II. Series.
  GV711.5.Y33 1994   94-18672
  613.7'11--dc20   CIP

ISBN: 0-87322-770-0

Developmental Editor: Holly Gilly; **Assistant Editors:** Ed Giles, Julie Lancaster, Dawn Roselund, and Jennifer Wilson; **Copyeditor:** Anthony Brown; **Proofreader:** Jim Burns; **Indexer:** Sheila Ary; **Production Manager:** Kris Ding; **Typesetter:** Ruby Zimmerman; **Text Designer:** Keith Blomberg; **Layout Artist:** Stuart Cartwright; **Photo Editor:** Karen Maier; **Cover Designer:** Jack Davis; **Photographer (cover):** © F-Stock/John Laptad; **Photographer (principal interior):** Zehr Photography; **Models:** Stuart Cartwright and Peg Olson; **Illustrators:** Tim Offenstein and Gretchen Walters; **Printer:** Bang Printing

Human Kinetics books are available at special discounts for bulk purchase. Special editions or book excerpts can also be created to specification. For details, contact the Special Sales Manager at Human Kinetics.

Printed in the United States of America   10 9 8 7 6 5 4 3 2 1

Human Kinetics
P.O. Box 5076, Champaign, IL 61825-5076
1-800-747-4457

Canada: Human Kinetics, Box 24040, Windsor, ON N8Y 4Y9
1-800-465-7301 (in Canada only)

Europe: Human Kinetics, P.O. Box IW14, Leeds LS16 6TR, England
(44) 532 781708

Australia: Human Kinetics, Unit 5, 32 Raglan Avenue,
Edwardstown 5039, South Australia
(08) 371 3755

New Zealand: Human Kinetics, P.O. Box 105-231, Auckland 1
(09) 309 2259

Contents

Part I   Preparing to Cross-Train   1

Chapter 1   Fitness Cross-Training   3
Chapter 2   Getting Equipped   13
Chapter 3   Checking Your Cross-Training Fitness Level   21
Chapter 4   Cross-Training the Right Way   29
Chapter 5   Warming Up and Cooling Down   35

Part II   Cross-Training Workout Zones   45

Chapter 6   Green Zone   49
Chapter 7   Blue Zone   63
Chapter 8   Purple Zone   75
Chapter 9   Yellow Zone   89
Chapter 10   Orange Zone   103
Chapter 11   Red Zone   117

Part III   Training by the Workout Zones   131

Chapter 12   Setting Up Your Own Program   133
Chapter 13   Multiple-Activity Workouts   143
Chapter 14   Charting Your Progress   151

Index   159

About the Author   163

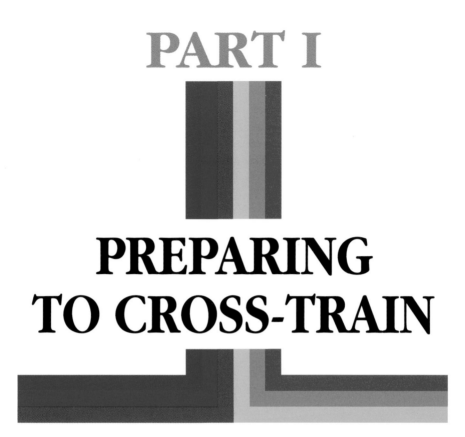

PART I

PREPARING
TO CROSS-TRAIN

Although hailed for its effect on the exercise psyche of exercisers and competitive athletes the world over, the amateur competition triathlon, which emerged in the 1970s, did not signal the beginning of cross-training. In the eyes of the exercise public, however, the term *cross-training* found a place in sports vernacular with the popularization of the biking, swimming, and running in the triathlon—a sport open to all who dared to try it.

Not surprisingly, decathletes, pentathletes, biathletes, rodeo cowboys, ski racers, all-around gymnasts, and a long list of other athletes knew cross-training not in theory but in practice long ago. Certainly, it was a necessary action to prepare their entire bodies and minds for competition. From their sometimes heroic efforts, including both successes (record-breaking times and dramatic victories) and failures (training injuries and disappointments), we've learned a great deal about training and performance, and today, it is yours for the taking. Throughout this book you'll be offered this information in a variety of ways.

A pivotal part of cross-training is preparation and planning. In the chapters that follow in Part I, we'll examine cross-training as an exercise program for developing fitness, and then we'll get you ready for cross-training by taking a look at your physical readiness and mental commitment, which includes costing out clothing and equipment needs for a multiactivity exercise program and having you take a personal inventory to check on your readiness for cross-training.

Chapter 1, "Cross-Training for Fitness," offers an in-depth look at the benefits of cross-training for athletes and fitness enthusiasts alike, with important distinctions made for each. This chapter explores the physical fitness potentials of cross-training, from cardiovascular conditioning to flexibility, as well as the importance of creating the kind of objectives that lead to an enduring cross-training program.

Chapter 2, "Getting Equipped to Cross-Train," looks at the kind of clothing, exercise gear, shoes, and the like needed to cross-train, with estimated price tags to assist your planning. In addition, this chapter provides special considerations and strategies for exercising in the elements.

In chapter 3, "Checking Your Cross-Training Fitness Level," there are self-tests to help you assess your readiness for cross-training and to determine the best level at which to begin. You'll also learn to take your pulse and calculate your target heart rate, and you'll take a self-test to assess and score your current fitness level.

Chapter 4, "Cross-Training the Right Way," delves more deeply into the actual mechanics and logistics of cross-training—when you can really begin to savor the fun and versatility of cross-training. Concepts explored include learning to select different exercise/sport activities to complement one another in meeting your fitness objectives; varying the mode, intensity, frequency, and duration of exercises to achieve desired results; understanding muscle specificity as it applies to cross-training; using key tips to make transitions between cross-training activities; and learning what to avoid when making these transitions.

Chapter 5, "Warming Up and Cooling Down," offers an excellent review of warming-up principles for cross-training and a number of specific flexibility stretches to use in your warm-ups and training routines. The chapter also explains the importance of a well-planned and correctly initiated cool-down, along with key stretching information.

Enjoy yourself! You've taken a big step forward with cross-training.

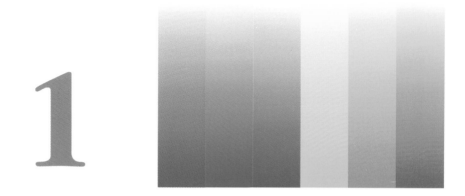

Fitness Cross-Training

If you want to discover more joy in exercising while exposing yourself to less risk of injury, fitness cross-training is for you! Cross-training is a strategy used by exercisers and competitors to organize their workouts and fitness activities, with the goal of providing as much variety and challenge as they need to stay on track in achieving their fitness goals in a safe and satisfying way.

A competitive cyclist, runner, swimmer, or skier might mix and match specific exercises and activities to train various body systems and body parts. These multiple training activities will ultimately make the athlete more proficient at his or her chosen sport.

In every instance, cross-training includes planned days of rest. A variable mixture of workout intensities is also used to encourage sustained overall improvement. So while some muscle-tendon-joint complexes are put to work, others are allowed to rest and recover, and while these parts of the body are recovering, the heart and lungs (as well as other body parts) may be working during another activity.

Because cross-training is so effective and flexible in its application, it is embraced by the broadest range of fitness enthusiasts and athletes: beginning exercisers, health club members, aspiring competitors, amateur and professional athletes. And the number of people doing some form of

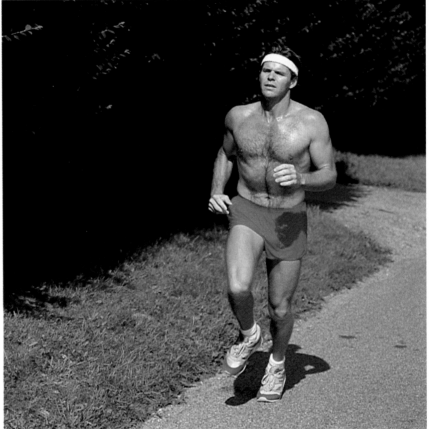

© Fabricius-Taylor/Photo Network

Taking a long, slow run the day after a tough swimming workout challenges the muscles of the lower body while the muscles of the upper body rest.

cross-training is expected to grow by as much as 70% over the next 10 years. Even triathletes add an average of three sessions of cross-training to their weekly swim, bike, and run training regimens, much of it linking weight training with their workouts.

Who Can Benefit From Cross-Training?

If you want to achieve significant fitness gains and engage in a variety of sports in which skills, power, speed, flexibility, or endurance is essential to performance, you need to start cross-training. Competitive athletes and serious exercisers who cross-train can train harder and longer with less risk of injury because they have learned one of the most important training principles: Don't overwork the same muscle groups without allowing 24 to 48 hours of recovery between workouts.

Athletes and exercisers alike who train a minimum of 6 days a week acknowledge the importance of this training principle by using cross-training. On Day 1, a challenging lower body workout (like hill running) might be accompanied by a lower body flexibility workout (maybe a low-impact aerobic activity followed by a stretching routine) later in the day, or the next morning preceding an upper body workout (perhaps interval swimming).

Categories of Exerciser

I group people who exercise into three main categories: beginning/easy, frequent/moderate, competitive/intense.

- **Beginning/easy exercisers** exercise occasionally, or when it's convenient. Generally, their workouts are in the Green to Purple zones (easy to moderate intensity and short duration) and their workout routines are not "planned" (with each workout intended to complement another workout or series of workouts).
- **Frequent/moderate exercisers** tend to have exercise goals oriented to personal needs (weight control, waist control, leg toning, buttock firming, muscle building/sculpting), but these may not be uniformly integrated with other workouts to actually achieve these goals. They often use exercise to work out with others and because they know it's good to exercise regularly. (They're right—regular exercise is good for every body and every mind!) Workout intensity for these exercisers varies from low-moderate to low-high.
- **Competitive/intense exercisers** plan workouts that are intended to progress them toward a primary goal (often a specific performance marker like a completion time for an event, a height achieved, a distance traveled, a weight lifted, or competition finished). Each workout is intentionally connected to the next to build toward specific performance goals, and workouts are planned to create incremental progress over a week's or month's time (or longer). A progression of activities is planned to achieve long-term results, which may address personal needs as well as athletic/sport needs. Competitive/intense exercisers may be motivated at times by the social camaraderie in the exercise environment, although often for only competitive training reasons (which, as you'll read in chapter 4, may not always be as productive as intended).

Benefits of Cross-Training to Single-Sport Exercisers

Running. Runners can shorten the duration of fatigue in their legs after running by increasing flexibility in their legs and hips with activities like aerobics and swimming. Through abdominal cross-training they can stabilize their lower backs and midsections, improving uphill and down-

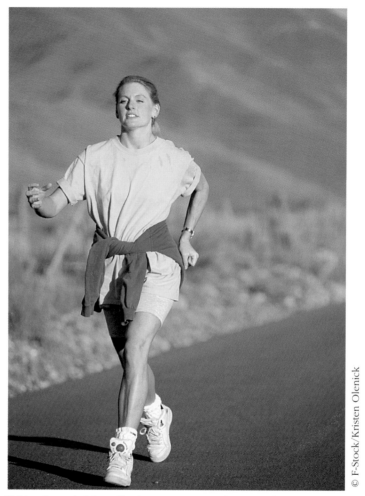

© F-Stock/Kristen Olenick

Taking long, brisk walks is one way exercisers can increase endurance.

hill running stride while adding to their potential for building endurance. Runners can also improve leg strength, lift, and power with weight training and build upper body strength for sprinting and racing with weight training and swimming.

Cycling.   Cyclists can achieve increased leg strength, speed, and power with weight training and related plyometric activity and can prevent low back problems with abdominal cross-training and aerobics. Running a long and slow distance will add to their endurance potential and cardiovascular development.

Aerobics. Aerobic exercisers can develop additional shape and tone from light-weight, high-repetition weight training, and can improve strength and stamina for aerobic strength moves and leaping movements from a more controlled power lifting regimen. Aerobic exercisers may increase endurance by adding periodic runs, long walks, and long-distance cycling or swimming. Chronic joint or muscle problems that may accompany exclusive aerobics (or running) may be mediated with complementary walking, swimming, or cycling workouts.

Swimming. Swimmers may add to their stroke versatility and power by developing their upper body strength and flexibility through a carefully constructed weight training program, and they may add to their muscular balance with regularly scheduled walks or runs. A low-impact aerobics class offers a contrasting stress, also known as a positive challenge, to swimmers' shoulder muscles, tendons, and joints. Weight training, cycling, walking, running, and aerobics may add leg strength that can be translated into a stronger kick. However, without key foot/ankle flexibility, the leg endurance might not matter for the swimmer.

Weight Training. Weight trainers benefit from all cardiovascular building activities that do not adversely tax those muscles and muscle systems they are training for a specific size or shape. Weight trainers increase flexibility from routine low-impact aerobics classes, and they may also use a variety of swim strokes at an easy pace without losing any weight training benefits.

Walking. Walkers may use weight training to develop a faster, more upright gait and to accentuate the leg strength gains they get from walking. They may use swimming or aerobics to counterbalance overall flexibility gains, particularly in the hips and midsection. Like runners and cyclists, walkers may use abdominal cross-training to further stabilize their midsections and to prevent low-back problems caused by abdominal weakness. Race walkers may use aerobics for flexibility and weight training to increase upper body strength and arm speed.

Fitness Components of Cross-Training

Clearly, no single activity provides full fitness benefits, and even the best miss the mark for persons with multiple fitness needs. Frankly, all athletes have multiple fitness needs, as do all serious and recreational exercisers. You need to recognize these myriad needs early on in the planning and design of your exercise program, because a poor training program design leads to chronic, even debilitating injuries.

Although analyzing the full range of activities for their fitness benefits is ill-suited to a book of this scope, there are some basic elements considered germane to overall fitness: cardiovascular fitness, muscular strength, muscular endurance, body composition, and flexibility. Understanding these as they apply to activity and training will better prepare you to analyze prospective exercises or activities in which you intend to engage (see Figure 1.1). If all of these elements are present in your exercise program, you will be focused on overall fitness.

Cardiovascular Fitness

There are four building principles of cardiovascular fitness: the type of activity you choose, how long per session you do it, how hard you perform the activity, and how often you do it. Although methods of achieving cardiovascular benefit are debatable, cardiovascular training should be an essential component of your exercise regimen, because it heightens the body's ability to transport oxygen to the working muscles.

Applying these principles, you develop cardiovascular fitness by regularly performing (3-5 times a week) activities that will raise your heart rate 60% to 80% of your maximum heart rate for at least 20 minutes. Generally, the more intensely you exercise for the appropriate durations and frequencies, the sooner the cardiovascular benefit develops. However, you won't maintain the cardiovascular benefits you achieve from high intensity workouts without continuing regular high intensity workouts.

Most exercisers work out at moderate levels of intensity, yet develop highly satisfactory levels of cardiovascular health by increasing the duration and frequency of their workouts. The majority of exercisers rely on one or two activities for successfully achieving a training heart rate. Cross-trainers, on the other hand, can choose from many options for their cardiovascular training.

Cross-trainers often look at their resting heart rate (RHR) as a measure of their level of cardiovascular fitness. RHRs vary among individuals, from as low as 38 to 45 for endurance athletes to 45 to 55 beats per minute for generally fit cross-trainers.

To determine your resting heart rate, first find your pulse by pressing your fingertips to the side of your wrist or the side of your neck under the jawbone where your voice box is. Count the number of pulses for 15 seconds and multiply by 4. Do this several times during the day to arrive at a good average for your resting heart rate. You can use this same procedure to measure your heart rate during exercise. However, people with heart and circulatory problems should consult with their physicians to establish reasonable values for their resting and exercising heart rates.

Muscular Strength

The strength of your muscles represents a ceiling, as it were, to your potential for explosive exertion, as well as a coat of armor for your

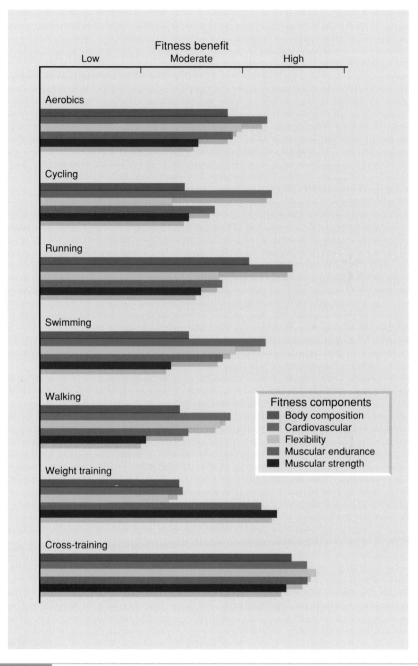

Figure 1.1 Fitness activities.

musculoskeletal structure and your vital body organs when at rest and during minimum to maximum exertion. Muscular strength enables you to approach varied training challenges with confidence and control. Clearly, the more broadly and systematically you challenge different muscles and muscle groups through properly planned cross-training programs, the greater your overall body strength and resistance to muscle-tendon-joint injury. You might be surprised that added muscular strength provides "acquired immunity" to everyday aches and pains. And with additional strength you'll be less susceptible to common muscle-tendon injuries from lifting, reaching, and throwing.

Muscular Endurance

To maximize your muscular strength in achieving broad fitness goals, it's important to train your muscles to remain strong during repeated use. To extract the greatest benefit from trained muscles, you must not only strengthen them but also train them *specifically*—just as they are to be used when you demand top performance. Triathletes are a good example of this concept as it applies to cross-training. For example, the muscular endurance needed to swim 2.4 miles is of little benefit to someone who is charging through a 112-mile bike ride and then lacing up for a 26.2-mile run. These distances are, of course, those of the Ironman Triathlon. Even the more popular international tri-formula of a 1-mile swim, a 25-mile bike ride, and a 6-mile run points to the same conclusion. Muscular endurance is achieved differently for the swim, the bike, and the run. I also believe in training for the transitions between each.

You develop muscular endurance the same way that you develop cardiovascular endurance, and depending on your sports or fitness needs, the level of muscular endurance you require will dictate how aggressively you must cross-train to develop it. Cross-training for the development of muscular endurance is preferred, because the variety of activities will tend to protect you from overemphasizing the development of certain muscles over others (see Figure 1.2).

Body Composition

The percent body fat to lean body mass (e.g., muscles and bones) is a critical measure of overall fitness. Body composition is a barometer of one's ability to balance the number of calories consumed with the number used while remaining cognizant of the nature of the calories consumed. Body fat plays a vital role in the functioning of many body systems, but excess fat is not only unhealthy, it also hinders one's ability to exercise and perform in sports.

What's the minimum percent body fat that's needed? For adult men it's right around 5% and for adult women, about 12%. An acceptable range of

	Running	Swimming	Cycling	Walking
Quadriceps	■		■	■
Hamstrings	■			■
Calf	■	■	■	■
Ankle	■			■
Buttocks	■		■	■
Hip flexors	■	■	■	■
Shoulder		■		
Chest		■		
Forearm		■	■	
Upper back		■		
Triceps		■		

Note: The legs and lower body benefit most from aerobics. Additional benefits are upper body toning and overall body flexibility. Specific muscle benefits from weight training depend on the training regimen. Weight training may provide strength, power, size, endurance, and tone.

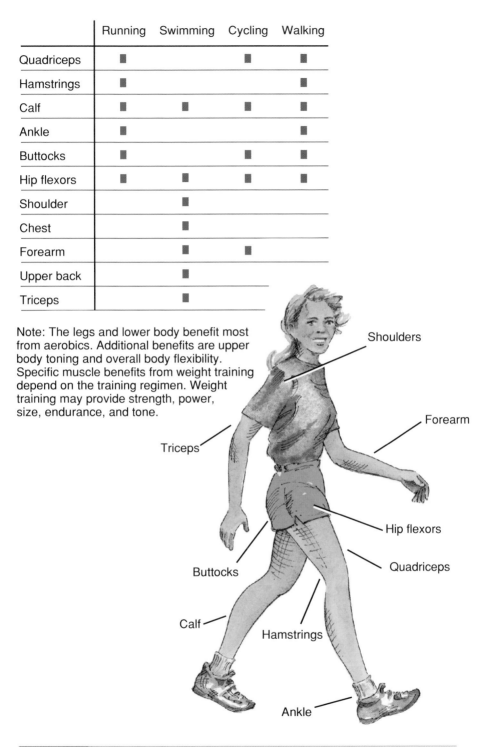

Shoulders

Forearm

Triceps

Hip flexors

Buttocks

Quadriceps

Calf

Hamstrings

Ankle

Figure 1.2 Muscle groups benefiting from different activities.

body fat is a relative concept. Physiologically, 5% to 20% is acceptable for men—although for male athletes (depending on the sport) this figure may be 5% to 15%. For women, 12% to 30% may be physiologically acceptable, but for female athletes (depending on the sport) the range may be 8% to 18%.

Excess fat adds stress to muscle-tendon-joint complexes and creates extra mass to manipulate. Put simply, extra fat makes it harder to move and increases the likelihood of injury when movement occurs. Although excess fat creates buoyancy while swimming, it's not necessary for long-distance swimming success, nor is it common among the top-finishing swimmers.

A steady course of endurance training is particularly effective in reducing body fat, because it improves the ability of muscles to use oxygen and to burn fuel more efficiently. By cross-training, you can do endurance training daily without the risk of injury from overuse.

Flexibility

Flexibility is the ability of skeletal muscles and joints to move through their full range of motion. As persons age, particularly men, flexibility gradually decreases, noticeably so after age 30. To increase or to maintain your present level of flexibility, it is essential that you properly stretch your muscles and tendons. You will find instructions for stretching in chapter 5.

Another passive means of flexibility is a cross-training program in which the demands on your muscle-tendon-joint systems are appropriately planned. For example, muscle-shortening and concentrated-muscle activities are followed the same or next day by muscle-lengthening or elastic-muscle-movement activities. Specific examples might involve running followed by swimming, cycling followed by aerobics, weight training followed by walking, and so on.

It's unfortunate that many exercisers and athletes don't stretch out before and after workouts. As a cross-trainer, you must stretch every time you train, either with specific stretches or with activities that employ movements that stretch muscles and tendons as part of their execution. Regardless of how advanced you become, refer to and use the information in chapter 5 often.

In the next chapter, I'll get you equipped for cross-training by reviewing clothing and equipment needs, costs, and training in various climatic conditions.

2

Getting Equipped

Cross-trainers are a sporting goods manager's dream come true. We could spend a fortune on all the shoes (at any given time of the year I own 10 pairs of exercise shoes, not including 4 pairs of ski/snowboarding boots), clothing, and equipment designed for specific fitness activities. What you will need to buy to get equipped for cross-training depends on your current stock of equipment and clothing, but before taking an inventory, consider the following safety and comfort guidelines.

Cross-Training Apparel

Apparel includes much more than clothing, and when cross-training it's important to identify all apparel vital to your overall training, such as shoes, gloves, eyewear, and headgear.

Shoes

Choosing the proper shoes is probably the most important decision you'll make in outfitting yourself for all but swimming. Shoes for running, walking, and aerobics, for example, should have at least the following:

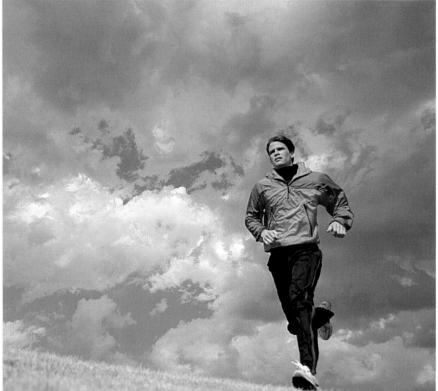

© R. Bossi

The most important piece of equipment for runners is a good pair of shoes.

- Internal and external PVC (polyvinylchloride) heel counters
- Correct arch support
- Correct fit and padding around the Achilles tendon
- Breathable material

In addition, running shoes should have an engineered outersole at the heel and midsole, and a tread pattern for your kind of running. Walking shoes should have cushioning for the instep, and the outersole should be flexible from heel to toe but should be rigid when twisted from side to side. In some of the cold regions of the world, "shoe chains" are used for training on snow.

Shoes for aerobics should have midfoot support straps to provide stabilization during lateral movements and a cantilever heel outersole for shock absorption. For cycling, you can use the same shoes that you use for running, walking, or aerobics (or any other activity you enjoy, such as tennis) if you have plain pedals. If your bike is equipped with a shoe/cleat system, you'll need cleated shoes. If you have toe clips, you should look for smooth-bottom shoes with high-abrasion tips and good lateral support for the forefoot.

Popular footgear training aids for swimmers include swim fins and "zoomers" (very short swim fins).

Gloves

Gloves are used to protect your hands from the cold while exercising outdoors, and to prevent calluses and blisters by cushioning your hands from the jarring effects of cycling long distances. Gloves also protect your hands from the corrugated surfaces on some weight training equipment.

Clothing

Not every activity has a stringent clothes requirement. However, padded shorts for cycling are most desirable for narrow-road bike saddles or seats, and for rough mountain biking. A riding jersey with pouch pockets is ideal for long rides. For cold weather running or cycling, cotton or lycra tights are an option, as are snug-fitting sweat pants.

Eyewear

Your eyewear needs vary according to your activities. For running, walking, and cycling use sunglasses or eye shields (goggles without the eye enclosure with the shield held on by a headband apparatus). Both should offer protection from harmful UVA and UVB radiation. Swim

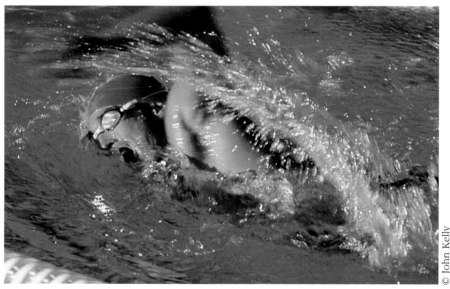

© John Kelly

Pool swimmers should always wear goggles.

goggles are essential for pool swimming, and most open-water swimmers prefer them as well, usually with shaded and smoked lenses.

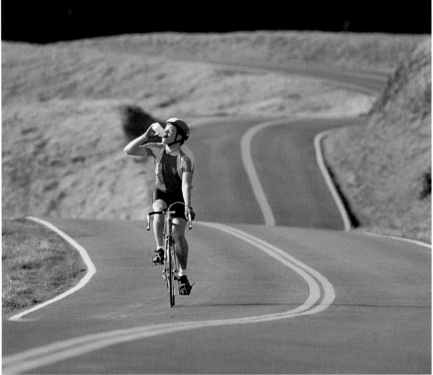

Always wear a helmet when cycling.

Headgear

The most significant piece of headgear is the bicycle helmet. It is a safety must! Runners and walkers may want to wear a cap or hat for cold or sun protection, and swimmers may wear a cap in the pool to decrease drag and to keep the chlorine out of the hair. Swimmers also may wear an insulated cap in cold open water.

Counting Up the Costs

Assuming a single year of cross-training with modestly priced and safe clothing and equipment, you can compare the costs of three different cross training programs:

Program One

This cross-trainer uses a program of smooth-surface cycling and running (no cross-country/trail running).

ITEM	COST
SHOES (2 PAIR):	$ 65 EA
SHORTS (2 OF EACH)	
CYCLING:	20 EA
NYLON:	13 EA
COTTON SOCKS (4 PAIR):	2 EA
RIDING JERSEY:	30
TANK TOP (2):	10 EA
RUNNING SWEATS:	25-80
RUNNING AND	
CYCLING TIGHTS:	12-25
RIDING JACKET:	25-50
ROAD BIKE:	350-800
AVERAGE COST:	$ 666-1,209

Program Two

Swimming, aerobics, and weight training are the chosen activities of our second trainer.

ITEM	COST
SHOES	
2 PAIR AEROBICS:	$ 50-75 EA
1 PAIR WEIGHT TRAINING:	35-60
ZOOMERS:	15
PADDLES:	8
GOGGLES:	7-34
SWIM SUIT (2):	20-40 EA
LEOTARD (3):	20-30 EA
SWIM CAP (2):	5 EA
TIGHTS:	20-30
GLOVES:	12

ITEM	COST
WEIGHT PANTS (2 PAIR):	10-20 EA
TANK TOP	
(2 FOR WEIGHT TRAINING):	13-20 EA
COTTON SOCKS (6 PAIR):	2 EA
WEIGHT BELT:	15-25
STUDIO/HEALTH CLUB FEES:	99-400 YR
AVERAGE COST:	$479-1,006

Program Three

Our last trainer likes a lot of variety, and trains by swimming, trail running or walking, cycling, aerobics, and weight training. Combining the costs from programs 1 and 2—less the costs of four pairs of socks, one pair of tights, and one pair of aerobic shoes—gives program 3 an average cost of $1,040 to $2,137.

Training in Different Climates and Conditions

There's a gymnastic club in Las Vegas, Nevada, whose slogan is "Go hard or go home." This sentiment holds true for serious and recreational cross-trainers, although the intensity with which each group exercises may vary considerably. Here's a rule of thumb for cross-trainers: If an exercise outcome is planned, then perform the needed exercise regardless of climatic conditions. Cross-trainers have an obvious advantage when dealing with changing weather conditions, because they have a menu of options from which to choose to achieve comparable exercise outcomes.

As you develop your own cross-training style, you will likewise develop a fairly reliable read on just what you may need to do to achieve your desired outcome. Given this fact, consider my generic guidelines for cross-training in varying climates and conditions:

1. **Foremost, plan for the weather by paying attention to the weather forecast and not by relying on your visual percep-tions of the day ahead.**

   In general, your level of activity will alter your body's experience of the weather by raising your body temperature. As your body temperature increases, the warm day will get hot or the cool day will get warm. Consequently, you must plan ahead for this eventuality. If you aren't prepared for the self-generated temperature change, you may find yourself uncomfortably overdressed, particularly on humid days. For

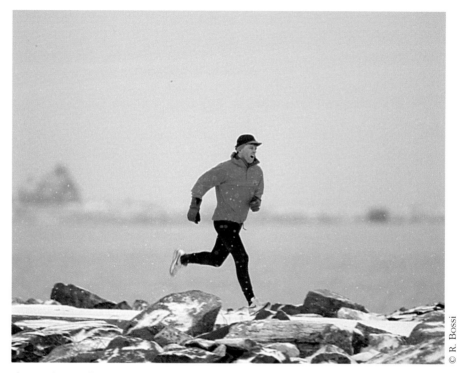

© R. Bossi

If you plan well, you can train in any weather.

example, cool winds may change a mild sunny day into a cold one and adversely impact your workout. Warm winds can affect your workout too by pumping up the day's temperature.

2. All training done outside is subject to relative risks. If it's the first rain of the season or the first after some weeks of dry weather, automobiles pose a relative risk to you if you use the streets for exercise. Riding a road bike in these conditions is ill-advised.

3. Exercising in the rain is no problem when the temperature is in the 50s and 60s, but I would advise you to wear water-resistant gear to prevent chafing.

4. Always anticipate risks to your safety when exercising outdoors. Risks can come from domestic and wild animals, motorized vehicles, bicycles, broken glass on the roadside, potholes, construction zones, and the like. On my runs over the years I've encountered bears, rattlesnakes, mountain lions, coyotes, abandoned mines, landslides, and even an earthquake!

5. When riding a bike, abide by the rules of the road; ride with traffic, and ride defensively.

6. When walking or running, sidewalks or roadside trails present the fewest problems. If running or walking on the edge of the road, face oncoming traffic and make eye contact with drivers at all intersections to make sure they see you. Consider the terrain before working out; rugged off-trail runs or hikes require correctly constructed running shoes or hiking boots.

7. Here are some special notes on cold, ice, and snow: You can dress in layers to stay warm and then peel them off as your body temperature rises. You may leave your extra clothes, once you've removed them, alongside the track or with a friend. You can also tie them around your waist or, depending on availability, check them into a locker. Ideally, plan ahead for where you are going to be exercising, and think about how you might deal with the need to add or subtract exercise wear.

   When ice and snow are present, you must weigh other considerations. Generally, ice is dangerous, and it's best to avoid it as a walking or running surface. Given the proper shoes and shoe coverings, 2 to 6 inches of snow make an excellent running or walking surface.

8. The time for which you schedule exercise determines the kind of adaptations you need to make. At dawn or dusk, reflective shoes and clothing are a necessity for exercising on the road. If walking at these hours, you should carry a flashlight to swing by your side as vehicles approach. If you exercise at midmorning, midafternoon, or at sunrise on sunny days, you may need sunglasses or a cap and visor to protect your eyes. At midday you may require other types of protection for your head or scalp.

9. When open-water swimming, paying attention to weather forecasts is critical. A mile out means a mile back to shore, and lake winds are notorious for their spontaneous occurrences—as are lightning storms.

10. Always be visually and audibly aware of what's going on around you. Anticipate other vehicles, even other exercisers, because either may do the unexpected. It happens all the time; cars have a blowout or swerve toward you, exercisers trip as you pass by, bikes skid out on sand or gravel, and people stop abruptly while walking or running. Always be aware!

In the next chapter, we'll check on your program readiness by looking at your fitness level, heart rate, and aptitude for cross-training.

3

Checking Your Cross-Training Fitness Level

Given all the knowledge today about fitness and sport, it makes little sense to fully engage yourself in any exercise or training program without first assessing your readiness for it. This chapter will help you take a look at your preparedness for cross-training and will then walk you through some self-tests to help you determine the kind of cross-training program that's suited to your level of fitness. The good news is that, regardless of the level of fitness, everyone has the ability to cross-train. Later in the book, I will provide programs suited to all levels of fitness.

However, first you need to examine the following Preparticipation Checklist to determine if you need to consult a physician before setting up your cross-training program. If you're honest with yourself when completing the checklist and when answering the questions in the tests that follow it, you'll be the benefactor of better planning and less injury. Again, I remind you that one of the distinct advantages of cross-training is that almost every exerciser, regardless of health status, can develop a program suited to his or her needs. However, you should consult a physician before beginning a cross-training program if you answer yes to any of the following questions.

PREPARTICIPATION CHECKLIST

	Yes	No
1. Do you have a history of heart disease, vascular disease, or blood clots?	___	___
2. Are you under the care of a physician for any heart or circulatory condition?	___	___
3. Do you have diabetes and take insulin to control it?	___	___
4. Do you take any daily medication that may be affected by exercise?	___	___
5. Are you over 45 and have you not exercised over the past 5 years?	___	___
6. Are you currently undergoing rehabilitation for an occupational or accident-related injury?	___	___
7. Do you smoke 10 or more cigarettes a day?	___	___
8. Is there a history of heart disease in your family, and have you not been exercising or exercising infrequently?	___	___
9. Have you noticed a shortness of breath or lightheadedness after any sustained aerobic exertion, such as riding a stationary bike for 20 or more minutes? (This does not apply to anaerobic exertion like sprinting or running up and down a basketball court.)	___	___
10. Do you have chronic orthopedic problems, arthritis, or other metabolic diseases?	___	___
11. Are you pregnant, and have you not been exercising prior to or at all during pregnancy?	___	___

Test Your Program Readiness

Because cross-training involves a nearly limitless selection of activities to round out your program, your test of readiness may vary considerably, depending on the nature of fitness you wish to achieve.

The following exercise is designed to help you interpret your cardio-vascular fitness and current readiness for a cross-training program. For each of the following questions choose the number that best describes your answer, using this scale: 3 (yes, a lot), 2 (occasionally), or 1 (no).

ASSESSING YOUR CROSS-TRAINING READINESS

Activity	Current readiness for a cross-training program
Do you run or jog?	_____
Do you swim?	_____
Do you cycle?	_____
Do you train with weights?	_____
Do you walk or hike briskly?	_____
Do you aerobic dance or aerobic exercise?	_____
Do you row or paddle?	_____
Do you rollerskate or in-line skate?	_____
Do you cross-country ski?	_____
Do you jump rope?	_____
Do you play soccer?	_____
Do you play racquet sports?	_____
Do you golf?	_____
Do you bowl?	_____
Do you play volleyball?	_____
Do you play basketball?	_____
Do you play baseball?	_____
Do you play flag or touch football?	_____
Subscore:	_____

Injury profile: **For this section, use the following scale: 1 (yes), 2 (sometimes), or 3 (rarely or never).**

Do you get foot or ankle injuries?	_____
Do you get upper body or shoulder injuries?	_____
Do you have lower back problems?	_____
Subscore:	_____

Weight status: **For this section, select one of the options. Your score is listed to the right.**

Are you within 10 pounds of your ideal weight? _____ (3)

Are you 11 to 19 pounds over or under your ideal
   weight? _____ (2)

Are you 20 pounds or more over or under your
   ideal weight? _____ (1)

   Subscore: _____

Pulse status: **For this section, select one of the options. Your score is listed to the right.**

Is your resting pulse below 60 beats per minute? _____ (4)

Is your resting pulse 60 to 69 beats per minute? _____ (3)

Is your resting pulse 70 to 75 beats per minute? _____ (2)

Is your resting pulse 76 or more beats per minute? _____ (1)

   Subscore: _____

Cardiovascular history: **What is your heart history? For this section, select one of the options. Your score is listed to the right.**

No history of heart or circulatory problems? _____ (3)

Past conditions now treated and reversed? _____ (2)

Heart and circulatory problems self-monitored? _____ (1)

   Subscore: _____

Smoking status: **For this section, select one of the options. Your score is listed to the right.**

Do you smoke at least 10 cigarettes a day? _____ (1)

Do you sometimes smoke? _____ (2)

Do you never smoke, or have you quit at least
   12 months ago? _____ (3)

   Subscore: _____

Total score: _____

After determining your total score, use the following scales to interpret the scores:

58-79 = You have excellent readiness for cardiovascular and sports performance cross-training.

39-57 = You need to exercise caution in your planning of activities, but do plan a program.

26-38 = It's best to seek professional advice and assistance in planning your program.

Finding Your Target Heart Rate

A basic tenet of training is to use your heart rate, the number of beats per minute, to monitor your exertion so that you train hard enough to achieve gains yet not so hard as to exceed your given needs. The purpose of an activity is to reach your target heart rate and to maintain it for 20 to 40 or more minutes, before gradually exiting the activity.

As a fitness-assessment bonus, your resting heart rate also suggests your level of fitness; the lower your resting heart rate (given no history of an abnormally low heart rate independent of exercise training), the more fit you are.

Your target heart rate will vary depending on your fitness and training goals. Generally, working within 55% to 75% of one's maximum heart rate is an athletic training range while 40% to 50% might be more ideal for sustaining weight loss and 75% to 90% more suited to serious athletic or competitive training. In other words, your training heart rate is a percentage of your estimated maximum heart rate.

To determine your maximum heart rate, subtract your age from the number 220. So if you're 35 years old, your maximum heart rate would be estimated to be 220 – 35, or 185. To determine any level of training heart rate, simply multiply 185 by the percentage you seek. A training heart rate of 70% would be 185 × .70, or 129.5 (130).

To use this information, you must be able to quickly and efficiently take your pulse, or heart rate. Although it's easy to do, a little practice increases the validity of each effort.

To take your pulse, place the pads of your index and middle fingers on the underside of your wrist just below the thumb and feel for your pulse. Using the same fingers, you may also want to try to check your pulse on the side of your neck between your chin and your Adam's apple. In either case, feel for the pulse and count the beats for 15 seconds, then multiply by 4 to determine your heart rate per minute.

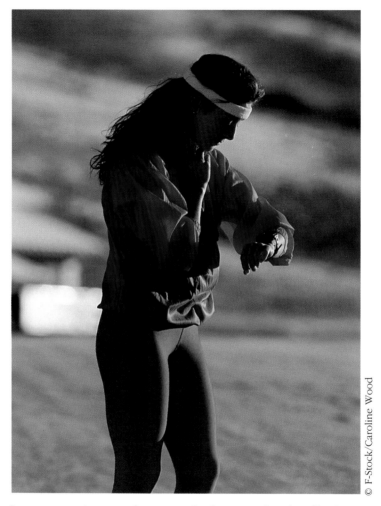

© F-Stock/Caroline Wood

Some cross-trainers use heart rate checks to monitor the effectiveness of their training.

Although I think it's wise to know your resting and training heart rates,
you may be like countless other recreational exercisers who view exercise
as a pleasant, nurturing activity; you may not be interested in heart rate
numbers, nor in taking your pulse during all aerobic exercise sessions.
Nevertheless, you do need to be aware of your body's acceptance of and
resistance to activity. You can monitor your efforts successfully by
employing a *rating of perceived exertion* (RPE).

With *perceived exertion* you should tune into your exercise in an
evaluative way by focusing attention to every part of your body and
determining what's going on within you in response to the activity. In a

very real sense, you become the expert on deciding when something is too much. You know when it's time to back off or to "rev it up" to keep yourself on course with the exercise.

Swedish physiologist Gunnar Borg identified a scale for individuals to use to determine their RPE. Originally, the scale included a numerical range of 6 to 20. Modified, the Borg scale of RPE has a numerical range of 0 to 10, with 0 being nothing at all, 0.5 being very, very light, 1 being very light, 2 being light or weak, 3 being moderate, 4 being somewhat hard, 5 being heavy or strong, 7 being very heavy, and 10 being very, very heavy (almost maximum).

The RPE will be used in this book to describe the level of exertion targeted in each of the 60 workouts in Part II. RPE values also parallel training heart rate ranges while exercising. For example, a beginning or easy exerciser may have an RPE of 2 to 3, with a corresponding heart rate of 60% to 69% of the maximum. A frequent or moderate exerciser may have an RPE of 4 to 5, with a corresponding heart rate of 70% to 79% of the maximum, while a competitive or intense exerciser may have an RPE of 6 to 8, with a corresponding heart rate of 80% to 95% of the maximum. A person exercising purely to lose weight may have an RPE of 1 to 2 and a heart rate of 40% to 59%.

Now that you've gotten a taste of the multidimensional scope of cross-training in the first three chapters, I'll begin to examine the nuts and bolts of planning and executing cross-training programs correctly and safely, which will further prepare you for the warm-up and stretches in chapter 5 and the cross-training zones in Part II.

Cross-Training the Right Way

Now you can really begin to savor the fun and versatility of cross-training. You're now on the path to becoming skilled at many activities, and as you progress in skill, you'll find that your appetite for other activities is robust. In fact, you may well overcome the barrier that holds back many exercisers from adding to their repertoire—the fear that they will fail to learn a new skill, sport, or exercise activity.

I will present a number of essentials for a productive cross-training program in this chapter: learning to select different exercise or sport activities to complement one another in meeting your fitness objectives; muscle specificity and exercise transitions; varying the mode, intensity, frequency and duration of exercises to help in your transitions; key mechanical tips for making transitions between exercises during cross-training; and highlights of mechanical errors in these transitions.

Effectively Mixing Workouts

If you are using only running and weight training in your workouts, let me give you a couple of examples of using these to complement each other.

If you wanted to develop speed and strength in your legs, you might mix three days of leg-focused weight training for power, while concentrating on variable-distance interval workouts (50, 100, 150 meters or yards) for two days and short sprints (40s and 60s) for one day. If you think your legs are getting too bulky, you could complement the weight training portion with a kickboard workout in the pool, during which you rest your forearms on the kickboard and kick continuously at a certain pace for 10, 15, 20, or more minutes.

If you wanted to develop more cardiovascular endurance, you could complement your long-distance running with a weight training routine that will build leg endurance and stamina with very high repetitions of relatively light to moderate weight. Essentially, if you're going to use exercises in a complementary fashion, you must first know your training needs and the potential benefits of different exercises.

Muscle Specificity and Exercise Transitions

One of the most annoying aspects of cross-training for newcomers is the sometimes uncomfortable transition between two very biomechanically different exercises. The complaints frequently heard are of sore muscles and aching joints, but both are preventable to a large extent by planning

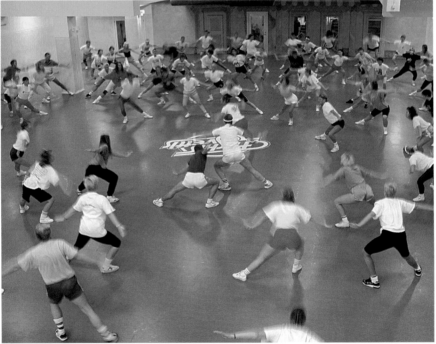

© Chad Ehlers/Photo Network

If aerobics is a new activity in your cross-training program, make a smooth transition by taking easy classes to begin with.

regular flexibility training and by respecting the concept of muscle specificity. Muscle specificity means that muscles are conditioned to respond to the demands they are given during habitual training. In other words, your muscles learn to do what they're trained to do.

Look at the demands of different exercises on your muscle system. At first, select those activities that have common muscle-use connections, yet that provide independent benefit. For example, the combinations of stairclimbing and cycling, walking and treadmill running, rope jumping and racquet sports, swimming and weight training, and even basketball, volleyball, and tennis all have their respective muscle-use connections.

Next, create a program of regular stretching to maximize the range of motion in muscles, tendons, and joints. (Use those stretches provided in chapter 5 and other appropriate stretches.) The added flexibility as a result of stretching will allow your muscles and tendons to "change gears" between exercises and thereby adjust and adapt to new movement patterns.

For example, if leg muscles are trained to run long distances at pace, they will get sore after a morning of running sprints, because long-distance running and sprinting make very different muscular demands. The same is true for a tennis player who starts playing soccer for cardiovascular training; sore legs will be the result a day or two later (usually the second day is worse).

The way to decrease the soreness following the introduction of new activities into your workout routine is to plan incremental transitions between activities within a single workout, between morning and afternoon, and from day to day. Chapter 13 has examples of multiactivity workouts you may want to try.

Help Your Transitions by Varying Mode, Intensity, Frequency, and Duration

When new exercises involve entirely new muscle systems, do not perform them to the point of fatigue or of even breaking a sweat. Plan three exercise sessions of transition where you increase the level of intensity and duration to allow your body time to adjust to and accommodate the new movements. I recommend these transition sessions be repeated for 3 days in a row. The Transition Tips on pages 32 and 33 will give you three examples of how to appropriately change from one activity to another during a workout.

TRANSITION TIPS

Swimming to Upper Body Weight Training

1. For every 30 minutes of swimming, allow 10 minutes of recovery before lifting weights.
2. Thoroughly stretch the shoulders, upper back, and neck immediately after swimming. Dry off and dress for lifting. Don't enter the weight room with wet clothes (yes, it happens); don't begin lifting without first gradually stretching; and when stretching, avoid ballistic or bouncing stretches, like jumping jacks.
3. Begin lifting immediately after the recovery, making sure shoulders are loose and relaxed.
4. Begin with general resistance exercises/lifts concentrating on the arms and shoulders, followed by heavier resistance for the chest, shoulders, and upper back. Conclude the weight training with exercises for the triceps, biceps, and forearms. Don't begin with heavy weights, and never attempt maximum lifts at any time after swimming.

Cycling to Running

1. Take off your helmet as you walk, taking long strides for a minute or two when you get off the bike, and then change shoes (definitely change shoes and socks—you're not competing).
2. Take off your gloves while you shake out your legs as if you're trying to keep someone from holding on to them. Avoid all ballistic toe-touching activities.
3. Be aware of any stiffness in your lower back, and pause to do standing arches as follows: Squeeze your abdominals, tighten your buttocks and lower back, and bow your midsection forward. Never assume you'll run through an aching back.
4. A shorts and top change is optional, depending on what you're wearing.
5. Begin running at an easy pace, lengthening your stride as you feel your hips and legs relax into the run. If your legs don't relax, stop to stretch your quadriceps, calves, and hamstrings. Don't begin running at full speed unless you are trained to do so.

Stairclimbing to Abdominal Work

1. Immediately after stairclimbing, stretch your Achilles tendons well. Make sure your stretch is held for an appropriate length of

time (10 to 20 seconds). Touching a heel briefly to the floor to each side is seriously insufficient.

2. Prepare your floor area for abdominal work, and stretch your hamstrings, calves, and lower spine before beginning abdominal floor work. Caution: Ballistic stretches risk injury.

3. If using abdominal machines or cable weights, stretch according to the previous tips.

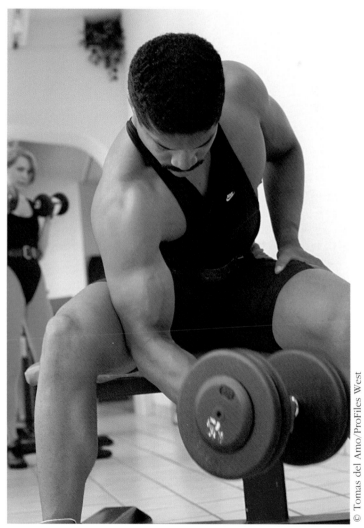

Using good lifting form is essential to avoiding injury.

After you've determined your body's readiness for any exercise or sport, you're ready to exert some control over the pacing of these activities to achieve your objectives. You do this by learning to vary your selection of the activity or *mode* most suited to what you feel you need, to regulate the *intensity* with which you do it (the more fit you are, the more you can crank it up), to determine the *frequency* or how often you need to do it to accomplish a desired effect, and finally, to establish the *duration* or how long you must do it to satisfy your body's fitness need.

As you advance in cross-training, you'll learn that the manipulation of mode, intensity, frequency, and duration of activity is central to controlling your progress and keeping injuries low.

Proper Mechanics and Form

The advantages of proper mechanics and form are many with respect to injury-free exercise and fitness gains, but less stated is the benefit of proper mechanics during transitions. In fact, most often it's the lack of proper mechanics and form in transitions that leads to injuries in novice cross-trainers.

Even so, remember that muscle specificity connotes regularity, and if you stop using a muscle system for weeks or months, you will encounter some degree of soreness when you return to the activity that works that muscle group. After any absence of activity, the transition to a once-familiar exercise requires attention to detail.

There's a lot to think about when first beginning cross-training. Developing an understanding of the basics is a huge stride forward. Now let's get warmed up and hit the road!

5

Warming Up
and
Cooling Down

Whether you're going to stick with one activity for an exercise session or engage in two or more, your potential to perform the initial activity and keep the risk of injury low depends a great deal on an *appropriate* warm-up.

Appropriate means you *never* go all out when beginning an activity, unless you have first engorged the working muscles with oxygen-rich blood, and it also means you use the warm-up time to take a personal exertion inventory.

Put simply, never go all out at first. Begin slowly and get the heart pumping blood to your muscles before any all-out activity. Going all out, whether lifting weights, walking, doing aerobics, skiing, cycling, swimming, or stretching, invites injury. And doing it habitually invites chronic injury, which plagues more than just the fitness element of your life.

A sound approach to warming up is doing a repetitive activity for 3 to 5 minutes that works your legs and upper body, coupled with appropriate stretching exercises or with a measured increase in tempo and intensity (like walking slowly for 3 to 5 minutes, building into a slow jog and then into an easy run).

Single-sport enthusiasts often benefit by inserting flexibility stretches into their warm-ups, though many will not. On the other hand, a well-conceived cross-training program will include flexibility as an integral component of training by routinely inserting flexibility stretches or by mixing and blending activities in such a way that they provide a natural "stretching" and relaxing of different muscles and muscle systems. A good cross-training program will promote flexibility in this way and make the physical transition between activities—for example, swimming and cycling—more fluid and comfortable.

Warming Up Is for Taking Stock

When you train regularly and plan a multiactivity exercise session or even when you've got a challenging single activity planned, your warm-up becomes a time of introspection and investigation. At a slow pace, you should assess the readiness of your body to meet the challenge you've planned by the way you're running, pedaling, or otherwise warming up.

I find this particularly important in training for triathlons and open and rough water swims. All three require that you exceed your comfort level physically and mentally, so it's important that you be in touch with your physical readiness. You don't want to attempt activities for which you're not prepared.

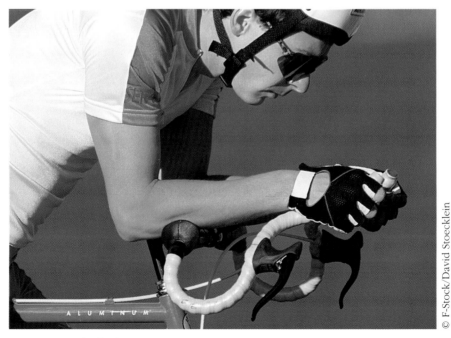

© F-Stock/David Stoecklein

Listen to your body during warm-up.

In short, warming up is a time to listen to your body: How do the legs, the shoulders, the chest, and the lower back feel? How's your breathing pattern? Is your swim stroke long or short? Is your running or walking gait lively or flat? What's your spin like on the bike?

Most importantly, you've got to learn how to listen to your body while exercising and then to trust what you detect. The slow-paced warm-up is an excellent method of developing this sensitivity. Going out fast blurs the body's caution signals and leads to injury, just as skiing fast often masks chronic problems with one's skiing.

The most significant training advantage of an appropriate warm-up is that it lets you use the results of your inventory to actually alter a planned workout. "Dead legs" may prompt you to change a planned long run to a paced cycling workout, a multikick-kickboard workout in the pool, or to deep water running with a flotation vest.

Warming up is not simply a convenient time to take such a personal exertion inventory; it's the *only* time!

Stretching Is a Strategy

Although you see a great many persons stretch a host of body parts before beginning an activity, unless the muscles and tendons are warmed up— that is, engorged with oxygen-rich blood and not warmed up as in a sauna or jacuzzi—the physical value of the stretching is questionable and may be very superficial. A good stretch follows shortly or immediately after the "engorgement" of the areas to be stretched, and it leads to gains in flexibility that benefit many other activities.

Again, the best way to warm up is to do something that steadily but easily works the large muscles in the body for 3 to 5 minutes while raising your heart rate. Walking, skipping, jogging, cycling, climbing stairs, dancing, and even rhythmic-standing leg or knee lifts all work to warm up your muscles-tendons prior to stretching.

Daily, moderate-intensity stretching is essential for healthy cross-training, particularly as persons reach 30 years old and over.

General Stretching Tips

1. **Don't bounce; press gradually, and hold for 10 to 20 seconds after you feel the tingling (but before the burning) sensation.**

2. **Use proper breathing by inhaling as you rest and exhaling as you press into the stretch.**

3. **Hold the stretches for 10 to 20 seconds. Gradually increase the length and duration of the stretches with each repetition.**

4. **Avoid weight-bearing stretches that keep your legs straight as you bend at the waist.**

5. **Deep knee bends, full squats, and lunges are not appropriate methods of stretching for flexibility.**

6. **Using weights as an aid to stretching is dangerous without careful supervision.**

7. **Effective stretches, those that produce flexibility, lengthen your muscles and tendons beyond their normal resting state, yet don't force body parts beyond their normal ranges of motion.**

On the next six pages you'll find 10 pre- and postexercise stretches that have broad applications to cross-training and are guaranteed to boost your flexibility and performance.

After you've developed your stretching routine, you'll notice significant improvements in flexibility within a few weeks. As you progress with cross-training, your ability to mix and match activities from the different workout zones that follow will open new fitness options for you and others who join your cross-training adventure.

Remember to hold each stretch once for 15 seconds, then a second time for 20 to 30 seconds.

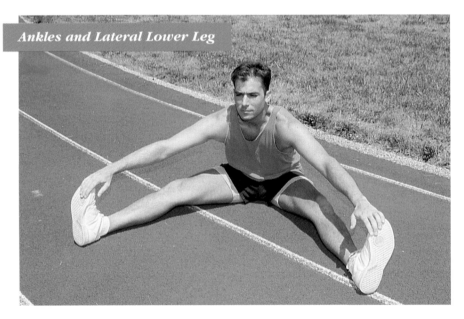

Ankles and Lateral Lower Leg

Sit upright with legs straight and straddled to the sides. Do not lock your knees. Slowly bend forward at the waist and grasp both feet while keeping the back straight. If you can't reach your feet, then wrap two towels around the bottoms of your feet and grasp the ends. Carefully turn both ankles inward. (This stretch helps prepare you for aerobics, running, walking, and aquatic exercises.)

Achilles Tendon and Posterior Lower Leg #1

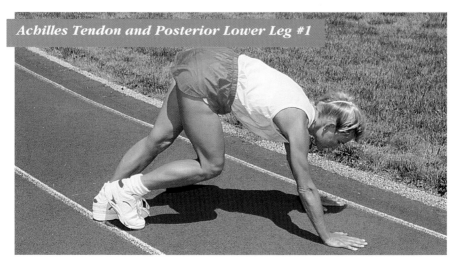

Place your body in a push-up position and slowly move your hands toward your feet until your body and the floor form a triangle. Carefully flex one knee and press your heel to the floor while keeping the other leg slightly bent. Alternate legs. *Note:* Do not bounce while doing this stretch. Keep motions slow and deliberate.

Achilles Tendon and Posterior Lower Leg #2

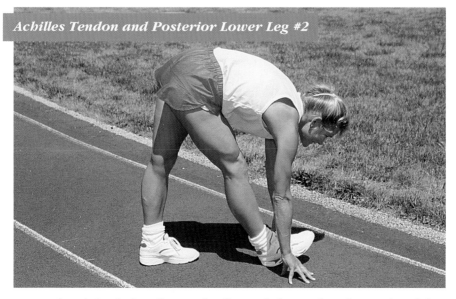

Stand with both feet flat on the floor. Shift one foot forward and flex your foot so your toes come off the floor. Gently bend forward and try to place your hands on the floor while keeping your back straight and your ankle flexed. Slowly return to an upright position and switch legs. (These stretches help prepare you for aerobics, running, walking, cycling, and aquatic exercises.)

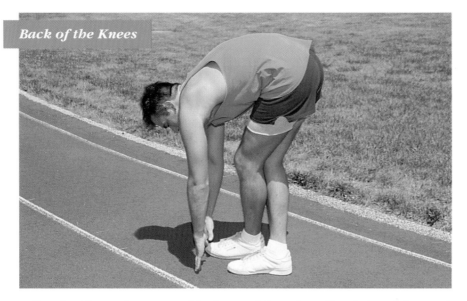

Back of the Knees

Stand with one leg crossed in front of the other. Slowly bend forward and reach toward the floor. Keep both legs fairly straight without locking either knee. Reach only until you feel a gentle stretch. Bend your knees and round your back to return to an upright position. *Note:* Do not perform this stretch if you have either back or knee problems. (Use this before running, walking, aerobics, and swimming.)

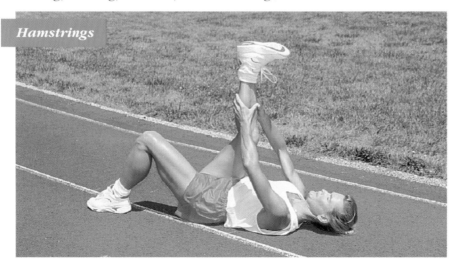

Hamstrings

Lie down with your feet flat on the floor and your knees bent. Raise one leg up and grasp it either below or above the knee—do not hold directly behind the knee. Gently pull your leg toward you until you feel a slight stretch. Switch legs. *Note:* Be sure to perform this stretch slowly and carefully, especially if you have back problems.

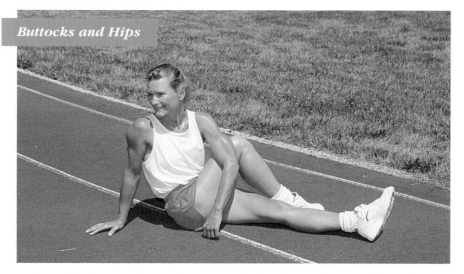

Buttocks and Hips

Sit on the floor with your legs extended in front of you and your hands behind you for support. Bend your right leg and cross it over your left, placing your right foot flat on the floor beside your left knee. Bend your left elbow and place it on the outside of your right knee. Push against the outside of your knee and twist your entire body gently to the right, trying to look backward over your right shoulder. Switch arm and leg positions and twist to the left. (Use this to prepare for running, walking, aerobics, and weight training.)

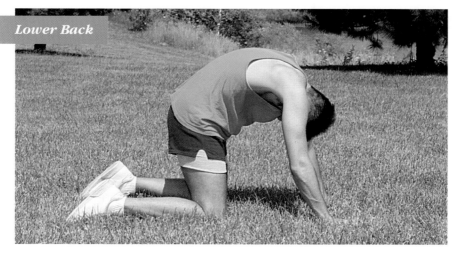

Lower Back

Kneel on all fours in a flat-back position while looking at the floor. Contract your abdominal muscles and tilt your pelvis under so that your back rounds up and forms an arch. Return to the flat-back position. (Use for weight training, walking, running, aerobics, and cycling.)

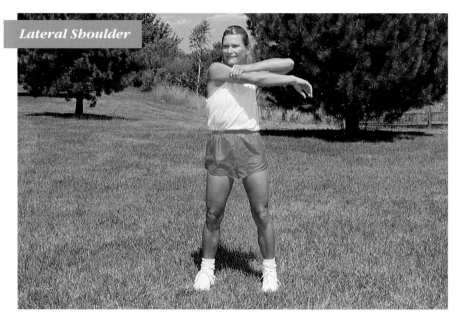

Lateral Shoulder

Stand with your right arm straight and raised to shoulder height. Reach across your body so your palm faces backward, and grasp your right arm with your left hand. Gently pull backward until you feel a stretch. Switch arms. (This stretch is good for swimming, aquatic exercise, and weight training.)

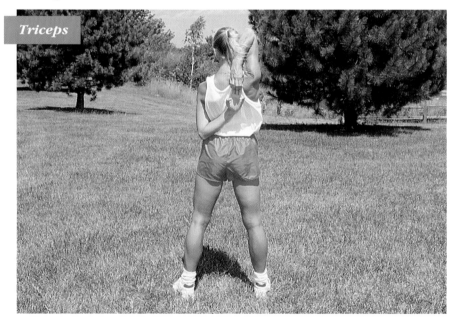

Triceps

Stand with your left arm raised overhead, then bend your elbow so your hand rests on your shoulder blade. Grasp your bent elbow with your right hand and gently push downward. Switch arms. (Use before swimming, aquatic exercise, weight training, and cycling.)

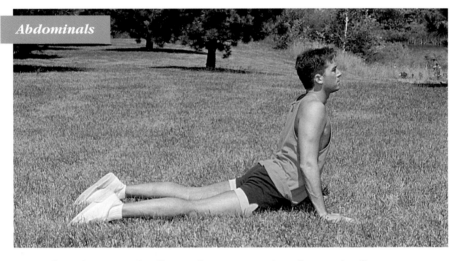

Abdominals

Lie face down on the floor. Place your palms flat on the floor near your hips (you may also use your forearms). Press down on the floor to raise your torso as far as you feel comfortable. Return to the floor. *Note:* Do not perform this stretch if you have back problems. (This stretch helps prepare you for weight training, walking, running, aerobics, and cycling.)

PART II

CROSS-TRAINING WORKOUT ZONES

The chapters in this part of the book use six different color-coded workout zones. The color-coded zones are designed to help you get a quick read on workouts appropriate for your current level of fitness, to help guide you in selecting workouts appropriate to meeting your overall fitness goals, and to accommodate your current training preferences and future training interests.

The Zones Defined

The workout zones are identified by *intensity* (training heart rate as a percentage of maximum heart rate) and *duration* (under or over 25 minutes). There are three levels of intensity addressed in these workouts: 60% to 75% of the maximum; 70% to 85%; and up to 100% of the maximum. Each intensity level has two varieties of duration (reflected in the color-coding), the first being under 25 minutes, the latter, over. The 25-minute mark refers to the time you are engaged in the primary activity, not including warm-up and cool-down times.

WORKOUT COLOR ZONES			
Zone (chapter)	Type of workout	RPE/ %MHR	Time
Green (6)	Low intensity, short duration	2-4/60-74	<25 min
Blue (7)	Low intensity, long duration	2-4/60-74	>25 min
Purple (8)	Moderate intensity, short duration	4-6/70-84	<25 min
Yellow (9)	Moderate intensity, long duration	4-6/70-84	>25 min
Orange (10)	High intensity, short duration	4-8/70-95	<25 min
Red (11)	High intensity, long duration	5-10/75-100	>25 min

The chapters that follow in this section include workouts for each of the following activities: running, swimming, fitness walking, aerobics, cycling, and weight training.

If you'd like to try a new activity, but you haven't a workout in mind, the range of intensity and duration will offer you a variety of choices to meet your needs in each of these six activity areas. In the third part of the book, I'll address these more in the context of creating cross-training programs to meet your needs.

At the end of each chapter in Part II, there's a section on how experts might use the workouts. I think you'll find this particularly instructive, because it gives you a sense of the scope of training strategies used by even the most well-trained competitive athletes.

As you read through the workout zone chapters, think about your workout choices, and make note of what you think the most appropriate workout zones are for your fitness level. Quite naturally, your workout zone for one activity may be entirely different from the others. Certainly, making exercise choices is one of the decision-making elements of fitness training that derails many well-intentioned exercisers. Bouncing around the workout zones will add variety to decision making and increase your adherence to training.

Overall, when you consider your workout choices, be honest with yourself in assessing the value and the suitability of the activity. Address the following:

- **Purpose.** What is the area of fitness you're hoping to improve—general training, speed and power, endurance, agility, flexibility, enhanced quality of sports performance? Does the workout offer the potential for you to achieve your purpose?
- **Participation.** What must be in place for you to perform the workout—the correct circumstances or logistics, the time of day, the need for a specific warm-up, for a coach or observer, for a competitor or comrade, or for specific equipment?
- **Practicality.** How may you continue to use this activity to advance or enhance your cross-training program and to keep you on track to meeting your personal fitness needs?

Caloric Cost

Part of the planning for fitness and well-being is calorie management, both from an input and output perspective. The focus of this book is on caloric output through exercise, and to this end, the calories burned during each of the 60 workouts in the following 6 chapters are calculated for you.

For perspective, your body uses 1 to 1-1/2 calories per minute to maintain basic body functions. As soon as you begin exercising, your body demands additional calories to fuel exercising muscles and to respond to its increased overall demand for energy.

Different exercises place variable caloric demands on your body. The level of exercise intensity, the person's body weight and relative muscle mass, the level of exercise efficiency, and the temperature in which one is working out influence the number of calories expended during an exercise session. As you might imagine, the caloric costs along the spectrum of workouts in this book will vary considerably.

Given the many factors that influence caloric cost, the best I can do is give you estimates of the number of calories burned. The estimates are based on the caloric cost for a person weighing 150 pounds. As a rule, for every 15 pounds above or below 150, you should add or subtract 10%, respectively, of the estimated number of calories burned for each workout. Thus, a workout that burns 300 calories for a person weighing 150 pounds would burn 330 calories for a person weighing 165 pounds and 270 calories for a person weighing 135 pounds. You must make these calculations as needed.

As an added guide to the caloric cost of the workouts in this part of the book, I have broken down for each of the six activities the average caloric cost per minute for a person weighing 150 pounds (see Table II.1). Warm-up and cool-down activities burn calories as well, although far fewer. Similarly, hill climbing in any of the activities adds caloric expenditure, as do speed, shorter recovery periods between exertion, increased resistance, and surges in intensity, also known as "spikes."

Table II.1
Caloric Cost of Workouts Per Workout Zone Kilocalories
per Minute/Kilocalories per Workout
(e.g., Green = 10/<250)

Activity	Green	Blue	Purple	Yellow	Orange	Red
Running	10/<250	10/>250	15/<375	15/>375	20/<500	20/>500
Swimming	7/<175	7/>175	11/<275	11/>275	14/<350	14/>350
Cycling	7/<175	7/>175	11/<275	11/>275	14/<350	14/>350
Walking	6/<150	5/>150	10/<250	10/>250	15/<375	15/>375
Aerobics	6/<150	6/>150	8/<200	8/>200	12/<300	12/>300
Weight training	4/<100	4/>100	6/<150	6/>150	9/<225	9/>225

Having assessed your readiness for cross-training and having planned appropriate fitness objectives, you'll be able to use the workouts in the following chapters to craft an exercise program that really works for you physically, emotionally, and socially!

Green Zone

Some persons think of easy as "wimpy," but in fitness training "easy" is a smart way to be tough. Even those fitness enthusiasts and athletes who work hard and long for a variety of personal and competitive reasons train easy at times, and most of them trained in the Green zone when they first began new workout activities.

Using Green Zone Workouts

Although Green zone workouts are sessions of their own, in cross-training they also serve as vehicles for you to integrate new workouts into your overall training; in effect, they are opportunities to try out new workout ideas and activities.

Green zone workouts may also be used as transitions during a multiactivity workout (where two or more activities comprise a single workout). As a rule, Green workouts raise your heart rate to 60% to 69% of your maximum heart rate and last less than 25 minutes. Sometimes transitional activities, like jogging or walking from the aerobics room to the weight room, from weightroom to pool, from fitness facility to an outdoor track, and so forth, are not workouts at all and are more properly labeled as very-low-intensity-workout transitions.

To sum it up, think of transitional activities as preparatory periods for the next challenge to your muscles, tendons, and joints. Linking relative rest to active preparation is one of the charms and challenges of cross-training, and at higher intensities, Green zone workouts serve as ideal transitions in a major training effort.

Two specific uses of the low-intensity, short-duration workouts are presented in this chapter:

- These workouts can introduce new activities into your cross-training program. At Green levels, you can get a feel for the new activity without excessive stress or postexercise soreness to your body.
- You can use Green workouts as a "training holiday" when you need to take a break from demanding workouts, yet still feel the need to do something of value.

WORKOUT 1

EASY RUN
TOTAL TIME: 25-30 minutes

1

WARM-UP: Walk 5 minutes at a comfortable pace, then break into the workout.

WORKOUT

Activity: Easy running or jogging on level terrain
Distance: 1-1/2 miles, but no more
Time: 15-20 minutes of easy jogging
Pace: 10- to 13-minute mile pace
Effort: RPE 2-3; % max heart rate 60-69

COOL-DOWN: Walk slowly for 3 minutes with an exaggerated arm swing that corresponds to your walking pace, then stretch for 5 minutes.

CALORIES BURNED: 150-200

COMMENTS

By breaking into easy runs out of a walk, you familiarize your body with the running motions. The arm swing helps release any upper body tightness. This workout can also be done on a treadmill.

WORKOUT 2

2

FUN TERRAIN RUN
TOTAL TIME: 30-35 minutes

WARM-UP: Walk 5 minutes on a level surface.

WORKOUT

Activity: Select a terrain site—a wooded trail, an open field, or a lawn area with uneven pitches—and run easy.

Distance: 1-1/2 miles

Time: 23–25 minutes

Pace: 13- to 15-minute mile; modify pace depending on terrain, with safety as your first consideration. Pace down for more difficult terrain.

Effort: RPE 2-3; % max heart rate 60-69

COOL-DOWN: Walk for 3 minutes and stretch for 10, concentrating on the hamstrings, calves, and ankles.

CALORIES BURNED: 230-250

COMMENTS

This is designed to challenge your dynamic balance, or your ability to adapt to out-of-balance sensations that are detected by your feet, legs, head, and eyes.

WORKOUT 3

SWIM DOUBLES
TOTAL TIME: 30-35 minutes

3

WARM-UP: A 60- to 75-second paced lap swim for 5 minutes, followed by a 3- to 5-minute stretch of your shoulders, triceps, and upper back.

WORKOUT

Activity: Swimming in 25-yard/meter pool

Distances: Yards or meters

Distance × reps	Rest* between reps	Rest* between distances
25 × 2	5 seconds	50 seconds
50 × 2	10 seconds	1:40
75 × 2	15 seconds	3:20
100 × 2	20 seconds	2:00 (before cool-down)

*Complete cessation of activity

Time: 15-20 minutes

Pace: At the beginning of the primary workout, each length of the pool should take 25 to 30 seconds; as distances increase, this time may also increase.

Effort: RPE 3-4; % max heart rate 60-74

COOL-DOWN: Easy swim—breaststroke or crawl for 3 to 5 minutes, and stretch.

CALORIES BURNED: 105-140

COMMENTS

Paced swimming assists your stroke development and prepares a new swimmer for more disciplined pool training.

WORKOUT 4

SWIM/PULL BUOY DOUBLES
TOTAL TIME: 25-30 minutes

WARM-UP: Easy 5-minute swim and 5-minute stretch.

WORKOUT

Activity: Like swim doubles, except on the second swim of each distance, you use a pull buoy and do not kick with your legs.

Distances: Yards or meters

Distance × reps	Rest* between reps	Rest* between distances
25 × 2	15 seconds	50 seconds
50 × 2	20 seconds	1:50
75 × 2	30 seconds	2:00 (before cool-down)

*Complete cessation of activity

Time: 15-20 minutes

Pace: 25-35 seconds per length

Effort: RPE 2-4; % max heart rate 60-74

COOL-DOWN: Easy swim with pull buoy for 100 yards or meters, and stretch.

CALORIES BURNED: 105-140

COMMENTS

Early in your exercise program, acquaint yourself with the use of a pull buoy, because it has many adaptations in future training. As long as your stroke is relaxed and efficient (your hands are completely pulled through), your overall exertion level is actually lower when using pull buoys, because you don't kick the legs. Moving the large muscles of the legs at a sprint pace is more taxing than moving only the smaller shoulder and arm muscles at the same pace.

WORKOUT 5

MILE RIDE × 2
TOTAL TIME: 20-30 minutes

WARM-UP: Ride for 5 minutes, pedaling in midgear range.

WORKOUT

Activity: Ride a measured mile in a high gear on a level surface. Stop for a brief stretch (2 minutes), and then ride the measured mile a second time in a low gear. Use high and low gear extremes to achieve the best results.

Distance: 2 miles

Time: 10-20 minutes

Pace: 6-12 miles per hour

Effort: RPE 2-3; % max heart rate 60-69

COOL-DOWN: Ride for five minutes in midgear range and do long body stretches and lower back arches to complete cool-down.

CALORIES BURNED: 70-140

COMMENTS

Experiment with a wide range of gears for the most benefit; you will notice the need for biomechanical adaptations to ride efficiently. For example, you may need to assume a more upright seated riding position in higher gears, or you may need to alter hand and arm position to accommodate changes in gears and demands on your lower body and back.

WORKOUT 6

6

EASY WALK
TOTAL TIME: 25-30 minutes

WARM-UP: Walk in place or walk slowly for 3 minutes. Lightly stretch for 2 minutes.

WORKOUT

Activity: Walking on level terrain or a treadmill with comfortable arm swing

Distance: 1 mile

Time: 15-20 minutes

Pace: 15- to 20-minute mile pace

Effort: RPE 2-3; % max heart rate 60-69

COOL-DOWN: Light stretching focused on your legs.

CALORIES BURNED: 90-120

COMMENTS

This is a casual exercise to lubricate the hip joints and to mildly tax the legs and heart, but it serves as an excellent activity if your spirits are down or if you can't do your planned workout.

WORKOUT 7

FUN TERRAIN WALK
TOTAL TIME: 30-35 minutes

WARM-UP: Walk on a level surface for 3 minutes, then stretch for 2 minutes.

WORKOUT

Activity: Select a terrain site—a wooded trail, an open field, a lawn area with uneven pitches—and walk easy.

Distance: Not relevant to the workout

Time: 15-20 minutes of continuous walking

Pace: Under 15-minute mile pace, but controlled for the terrain—seek challenges to your dynamic balance, such as gullies and ridges, boulders, and uneven paths, while maintaining pace.

Effort: RPE 2-4; % max heart rate 60-74

COOL-DOWN: Walk for 3 minutes, stretch for 5 to 10 minutes, concentrating on hamstrings, calves, and ankles.

CALORIES BURNED: 90-120

COMMENTS

Good for walkers who seek variety in their routines. Depending on terrain, maintaining your balance and pace may be a challenge.

WORKOUT 8

8

VIDEO AEROBICS
TOTAL TIME: 30 minutes

WARM-UP: Walk in place or walk around for 3 to 5 minutes. Stretch ankles, hips, calves, Achilles tendons, and hamstrings.

WORKOUT

Activity: Have the video aerobics tape cued to begin at a point that is 5 minutes before the aerobics section begins. Exercise to the tape for 15 minutes, 10 of which are in the aerobics section.

Distance: Not relevant to workout

Time: 15-20 minutes

Effort: RPE 3-4; % max heart rate 60-74

COOL-DOWN: Walk in place as you advance the tape to the cool-down section, and then complete the cool-down.

CALORIES BURNED: 90-120

COMMENTS

This variation of using aerobic videotapes allows you to use them more selectively, and it is a good opener to aerobics for the uninitiated. By using only a portion of a videotape, you can accentuate only that portion of an aerobic workout that best meets your immediate needs. This type of video workout is the only way some exercisers will ever try aerobics, so have fun with it!

WORKOUT 9

LOW-WEIGHT FAST CRUISE ON RESISTANCE MACHINES

TOTAL TIME: 30-35 minutes

9

WARM-UP: Ride a stationary bike for 12 minutes at a low level of intensity.

WORKOUT

Activity: Select a series of 6 to 12 fixed-resistance machines on which you can lift low weights repeatedly with little fatigue after 15 repetitions. Go through the series of machines using 20 repetitions for each exercise. Repeat two times.

Distance: Not relevant to the workout

Time: 15-20 minutes—during which you will go through the complete series using moderately paced repetitions. Aim for consistency in the lifting motion in both directions.

Effort: RPE 2-4; % max heart rate 60-74

COOL-DOWN: Floor stretches focusing on those muscles, tendons, and joints you worked on with the resistance machines.

CALORIES BURNED: 60-80

COMMENTS

A friendly introduction to resistance training, this is a muscle endurance workout and a good low-impact activity that has a measure of cardiovascular benefit.

WORKOUT 10

10

LOW-WEIGHT FAST CRUISE WITH DUMBBELLS
TOTAL TIME: 30-35 minutes

WARM-UP: Ride a stationary bike for 12 minutes at a low level of intensity.

WORKOUT

Activity: Use a series of 6 to 12 exercises that can be done quickly with low-weight dumbbells at repetitions of 15 to 20 per exercise. Repeat two times.

Distance: Not relevant to the workout

Time: 15-20 minutes

Effort: RPE 2-4; % max heart rate 60-74

COOL-DOWN: Use floor stretches that emphasize those muscles, tendons, and joints you've worked.

CALORIES BURNED: 60-80

COMMENTS

This is a muscle endurance workout and a good low-impact activity that leads to body toning and to some cardiovascular benefit. Proper form is a must when using any free weight.

How Experts Might Use These Workouts

Experts use Green zone workouts to provide

- a late-day workout after a morning race or competition;
- a leisurely workout for a mental holiday;
- an active-recovery workout following an intense session;
- a transition during an intense training session where a period of recovery is needed—but not as a break in the action;
- an active-recovery workout the day after an intense competition;
- an active period of recovery after an exercise-limiting injury;
- a safe alternative to working out an uninjured part of the body while other parts are injured (another of cross-training's charms); and
- an opportunity to try something different.

Experts like experimenting with Green zone workouts, because they are not physically demanding enough to "detrain" their muscle systems by reorienting them to the new, less demanding exercise. In other words, experts can maintain their muscle specificity in these workouts.

In the next chapter, you'll learn to take this introductory level of cross-training a step further by stretching out the workout time while maintaining a sensible pace with which to learn the proper biomechanics and technique.

Workout	Description	Duration (minutes)	Distance/Time	Intensity (RPE/% MHR)
		Summary Table		
		Green Zone Workouts		
1	Easy run	15-20	1-1/2 miles	2-3/60-69
2	Fun terrain run	23-25	1-1/2 miles	2-3/60-69
3	Swim doubles	15-20	Variable distances	3-4/60-74
4	Swim/pull buoy doubles	15-20	Variable distances	2-4/60-74
5	Mile ride × 2	10-20	2 miles	2-3/60-69
6	Easy walk	15-20	1 mile	2-3/60-69
7	Fun terrain walk	15-20	1–1-1/2 miles	2-4/60-74
8	Video aerobics	15-20	Partial tape play	3-4/60-74
9	Low-weight fast cruise on resistance machines	15-20	20 reps × 2	2-4/60-74
10	Low-weight fast cruise with dumbells	15-20	15-20 reps × 2	2-4/60-74

Blue Zone

While demands on your cardiovascular and musculoskeletal systems are generally low in Blue workouts, their longer duration permits a handsome portion of confidence building with respect to new activities you may want to incorporate into your training.

Using Blue Zone Workouts

Blue zone workouts may help boost confidence after an injury, because their low intensity accommodates a return to working out at a pace that's not likely to cause reinjury, yet is sufficiently long that the exerciser or athlete gets a "real" workout.

To be sure, the psychological effect on recovering exercisers and athletes of rating a workout as legitimate or as a joke should not be ignored. Blue zone workouts meet the test of legitimacy for both new and seasoned exercisers and athletes.

If weight management is a primary concern, you may want to focus on Blue zone workouts for their weight-loss potential. Research appears to show that long and slow training is one of the most efficient and least physically harmful ways to lose weight and keep it off, although there is growing evidence that carefully planned bouts of more explosive exertion may be used as a weight-loss strategy as well. Good weight-loss exercises will be noted in the workouts that follow in this chapter.

WORKOUT 1

1

TIMED LONG EASY RUN
TOTAL TIME: 45-50 minutes

WARM-UP: Walk 5 minutes at a comfortable pace, then break into workout.

WORKOUT

Activity: Running/jogging on level terrain
Distance: 3 miles, but no more
Time: 30-45 minutes of continuous easy jogging
Pace: 10- to 15-minute mile pace
Effort: RPE 3-4; % max heart rate 60-74

COOL-DOWN: Walk slowly for 5 minutes, then stretch for 5 minutes.

CALORIES BURNED: 300-450

COMMENTS

Consistent pace at low intensity is the theme here. This workout, which can also be done on a treadmill, is an important adjunct to a weight control program.

WORKOUT 2

LONG TERRAIN RUN
TOTAL TIME: 50 minutes to 1 hour

2

WARM-UP: Walk 5 minutes on a level surface.

WORKOUT
Activity: Select a terrain site (wooded trail, open field, lawn area with uneven pitches) and run easy.
Distance: 3 miles
Time: 35-45 minutes
Pace: 12- to 15-minute mile pace. Modify depending on terrain, but safety comes first; pace down for more difficult terrain. Distance is not the goal.
Effort: RPE 3-4; % max heart rate 60-74

COOL-DOWN: Walk for 5 minutes; stretch for 10 minutes, concentrating on the hamstrings, calves, and ankles.

CALORIES BURNED: 350-450

COMMENTS
Low-intensity terrain runs require the discipline to not get carried away and jaunt through the field (unless you've planned that and are in the physical condition for it) and to maintain pace.

WORKOUT 3

SWIM DOUBLES PLUS
TOTAL TIME: 45-50 minutes

WARM-UP: 60- to 75-second paced lap lane swim for 5 minutes, followed by a 5-minute stretch of your shoulders, triceps, and upper back.

WORKOUT

Activity: Swimming pool workout

Distances: Yards or meters

Distance × reps	Rest* between reps	Rest* between distances
25 × 2	5 seconds	50 seconds
100 × 1		50 seconds
50 × 2	10 seconds	1:40
100 × 1		1:40
75 × 2	15 seconds	3:20
100 × 2	30 seconds	2:00 (before cool-down)

*Complete cessation of activity

Time: 25-30 minutes

Pace: At the beginning, each length of the pool should take 25 to 30 seconds; as distances increase, this time may also increase.

Effort: RPE 3-4; % max heart rate 60-74

COOL-DOWN: Easy swim—breaststroke or crawl for 250 yards; stretch.

CALORIES BURNED: 175-210

COMMENTS

This workout prepares you to increase your intensity in the shorter distances as well as to increase your overall swimming endurance.

WORKOUT 4

SWIM/PULL BUOY DOUBLES PLUS
TOTAL TIME: 50 minutes to 1 hour

WARM-UP: Easy 5-minute swim and 5-minute stretch.

WORKOUT

Activity: Like swim doubles, only during the second swim of each distance and during the 100-yard swims between the distances, you use a pull buoy and use only your upper body for the swim.

Distances: Yards or meters

Distance × reps	Rest* between reps	Rest* between distances
25 × 2	15 seconds	50 seconds
100 × 1 (pull buoy)		50 seconds
50 × 2	20 seconds	1:50
100 × 1 (pull buoy)		1:50
75 × 2	30 seconds	2:00 (before cool-down)

*Complete cessation of activity

Time: 30-40 minutes

Pace: 25-30 seconds per length

Effort: RPE 3-4; % max heart rate 60-74

COOL-DOWN: Easy swim with pull buoy for 100 yards, then stretch.

CALORIES BURNED: 210-280

COMMENTS

Unless you swim at an easy pace, the workout will be more fatiguing than planned and may lead to shoulder joint injuries. Pace is an important training technique for swim training.

WORKOUT 5

5

MILE RIDE × 4
TOTAL TIME: 40-50 minutes

WARM-UP: Ride for 5 minutes, pedaling in middle gear range.

WORKOUT

Activity: Ride a measured mile in a high gear on a level surface. Stop for a brief stretch (2 minutes), then ride the measured mile a second time in a low gear. Use high and low gear extremes to achieve the best results. On the third ride, use your most comfortable gear and ride as fast as you can while maintaining pace—this is not sprinting! Do this again for the fourth mile.

Distance: 4 miles

Time: 25-40 minutes

Pace: 6-12 mph for first two and 15-20 mph for the second two

Effort: RPE 2-4; % max heart rate 60-74

COOL-DOWN: Ride for 5 minutes in middle gear range, and to complete cool-down, do long body stretches and lower back arches.

CALORIES BURNED: 175-280

COMMENTS

Remember, this is not a sprint workout (that will come soon enough), but rather one to establish pace control and riding efficiency.

WORKOUT 6

STATIONARY RIDE
TOTAL TIME: 52 minutes to 1 hour 12 minutes

6

WARM-UP: Do what is provided in the programmed exercise cycle; if the cycle is not computerized, ride easy for 5 minutes.

WORKOUT

Activity: Riding computerized or manual stationary exercise cycle

Distance: Not relevant to this workout

Time: 36-48 minutes of riding at a steady pace

Pace: To be determined by your comfort level; but should be between 70-80 RPM

Effort: RPE 3-4; % max heart rate 60-74

COOL-DOWN: Get off the cycle and stretch for 10 minutes after a few minutes of walking.

CALORIES BURNED: 252-336

COMMENTS

If you maintain proper pace, this workout is an aid to burning calories. Stationary cycles are particularly good for those days when you can't ride outdoors and you have a scheduled ride in your overall workout plans for the week.

WORKOUT 7

7

LONG EASY WALK
TOTAL TIME: 45 minutes to 1 hour

WARM-UP: Walk in place or walk slowly for 5 minutes; stretch for 5 minutes.

WORKOUT

Activity: Walking on level terrain or treadmill with comfortable arm swing

Distance: 3 miles

Time: 36-45 minutes

Pace: 12- to 15-minute mile pace

Effort: RPE 2-3; % max heart rate 60-69

COOL-DOWN: 5 to 10 minutes of concentrated stretching for your legs.

CALORIES BURNED: 216-270

COMMENTS

Long easy walks are beneficial for weight management as well as for general biomechanical conditioning for short runs and faster paced walking.

WORKOUT 8

ADVENTUROUS TERRAIN WALK
TOTAL TIME: 50 minutes to 1 hour

8

WARM-UP: Walk on a level surface for 3 minutes; stretch for 3 minutes.

WORKOUT

Activity: Select a terrain site—a wooded trail, an open field, a park—with numerous obstacles and changes in pitch. Pretend the negotiation of obstacles and pitch of terrain is an adventure—so choose your site accordingly. Walk easy, occasionally breaking into a slow jog for a short while, and then resume your walk.

Distance: 2-3 miles

Time: 35-40 minutes

Pace: Steady, under 15-minute mile pace, controlled for the terrain

Effort: RPE 2-3; % max heart rate 60-69

COOL-DOWN: Walk for 3 minutes, stretch for 10 minutes, concentrating on hamstrings, calves, and ankles.

CALORIES BURNED: 210-240

COMMENTS

Almost like hiking on variable terrain, this workout is intended to create a baseline for more challenging walking, which will help you achieve fitness gains.

WORKOUT 9

9

VIDEO AEROBICS
TOTAL TIME: 45 minutes to 1 hour

WARM-UP: Walk in place or walk around for 3 to 5 minutes. Stretch ankles, hips, calves, Achilles tendons, and hamstrings.

WORKOUT

Activity: Have a low-impact aerobics tape cued to begin at a point that is 5 minutes before the aerobics section begins. Exercise to the tape for 30 minutes with 15 to 20 minutes of it in the aerobics section.

Distance: Not relevant to this workout

Time: 30 minutes

Effort: RPE 3-4; % max heart rate 60-74

COOL-DOWN: Walk in place as you fast-forward the tape to the cool-down section, then complete the cool-down.

CALORIES BURNED: 180

COMMENTS

This variation of using aerobic video tapes enhances your overall exercise routine en route to meeting your specific fitness goals.

WORKOUT 10

LOW-WEIGHT SLOW CRUISE ON RESISTANCE MACHINES

10

TOTAL TIME: 45 minutes to 1 hour

WARM-UP: Easy ride on a stationary bike for 12 to 18 minutes.

WORKOUT

Activity: Select a series of 6 to 12 fixed-resistance machines, and using low weights that can be lifted repeatedly with little fatigue after 15 repetitions, go through the series of machines using 20 repetitions for each exercise. Repeat two times, using a consistent lifting motion in both directions.

Distance: Not relevant to this workout

Time: 30-40 minutes

Effort: RPE 3-4; % max heart rate: 60-74

COOL-DOWN: Floor stretches focusing on those muscles, tendons, and joints that were worked by the resistance machines.

CALORIES BURNED: 120-160

COMMENTS

You should develop a working relationship with fixed-weight-resistance machines. Slow deliberate movements are the product of discipline and patience—that is, a singular focus—and they will produce the changes you seek with weight training. This is the secret to success with these machines. Go through a complete series as outlined, using slowly paced repetitions (slow lifting demands a longer contraction of the muscle as well as a higher caloric demand), and you will increase the muscle-building demands on your body.

How Experts Might Use These Workouts

Here's how experts use Blue zone workouts:

- As much as two days after an intense endurance competition, experts consider a long and slow run or a paced mile or two-mile swim restorative and rejuvenating for otherwise stressed muscles, tendons, and joints.
- After a planned day off, a Blue zone walking workout or ride on the stationary bike may be a way to kick off a two-a-day workout for the beginning of a new training cycle for an upcoming competition.
- Blue zone workouts are used during recovery from competition-limiting injuries to maintain cardiovascular conditioning without taxing injured muscles, tendons, and joints.

In the next chapter, you'll take this expanded level of cross-training further by increasing the intensity another step, which will likewise increase your exercise and fitness options.

	Summary Table **Blue Zone Workouts**			
Workout	**Description**	**Duration (minutes)**	**Distance/Time**	**Intensity (RPE/% MHR)**
1	Timed long easy run	30-45	3 miles	3-4/60-74
2	Long terrain run	35-45	3 miles	3-4/60-74
3	Swim doubles plus	25-30	Variable distances	3-4/60-74
4	Swim/pull buoy doubles plus	30-40	Variable distances	3-4/60-74
5	Mile ride × 4	25-40	4 miles	2-4/60-74
6	Stationary ride	36-48	70-80 RPM	3-4/60-74
7	Long easy walk	36-45	3 miles	2-3/60-69
8	Adventurous terrain walk	35-40	2-3 miles	2-3/60-69
9	Video aerobics	30	Partial aerobic tape	3-4/60-74
10	Low-weight slow cruise on resistance machines	30-40	20 repetitions × 2	3-4/60-74

8

Purple Zone

Purple zone workouts raise your intensity to 70% of your maximum heart rate, but the duration will remain under 25 minutes. An often easier way for exercisers to make the transition to Purple zone workouts is by adding intensity boosters (like hills/inclines and steps/stairways) to familiar workouts.

Another tactic for manipulating intensity in your workouts is to add timed and variable aerobic and anaerobic phases to the workouts. Aerobic refers to a more consistent level of activity that tends to be longer in duration and that relies on a good heart and lung system to provide oxygen and nutrients to the working muscles. Anaerobic refers to shorter bursts of exertion, and explosiveness in your muscle activity.

Hills and steps have been added to many of the workouts that follow, as have aerobic and anaerobic phases. Think of these short-duration workouts as the component of cross-training that gives you the time to gain experience in using hills and steps while ensuring the opportunity to achieve greater mastery over workout planning.

As you venture more deeply into cross-training, you shouldn't think of your increasingly demanding workouts as harder but as more intense. It's all a mind game; if you think your workouts are getting harder, you're more likely to put off exercising, but if you think of them as more intense, you'll bring the challenge more into focus. Still, intensifying your workouts is not automatically beneficial, and in the next chapter I'll examine some of the potential pitfalls of increasing intensity without proper planning.

Using Purple Zone Workouts

Whether planning new workout routines for your cross-training regimen, testing your progress on learning new skills and activities, or wanting simply to "amp up" your workout, Purple zones are the ideal vehicle.

The beauty of Purple zone workouts is their flexibility and variety at those times when you're at developmental crossroads in your training. Use Purple zone workouts in these ways:

- Try altering your normal sequence of activities with the introduction or addition of a multiactivity, cardiovascular-building workout session.
- Test your crawl stroke learned in the pool with an open-water or timed pool swim of the appropriate length or time.
- Take one of your multiactivity Green zone workouts and convert it to Purple, and then do a subjective assessment of your performance at this level of intensity.

WORKOUT 1

UP AND DOWNHILL RUN
TOTAL TIME: 25-30 minutes

1

WARM-UP: Jog on a level surface for 5 minutes, followed by a brief 3-minute stretch.

WORKOUT

Activity: Use an incline you can run up and down. Ideally, use a 400-yard or meter section of trail, roadway, or sloping lawn. Run up the hill, pause for 10 seconds, and run down. Rest for as short a time as you need, and resume running up and down the hill. Every time you ascend the hill, add 5 seconds recovery time (for example, 10 + 5 + 5 + 5 . . .). Try to run the hill 3 to 4 times.

Distance: Variable 400-yard or 400-meter hill climbs and declines; could be 1,600 to 2,000 yards/meters total

Time: 10-12 minutes

Pace: Half-sprint

Effort: RPE 4-6; % max heart rate 70-84

COOL-DOWN: Walk halfway up the hill, then down, then stretch for 5 minutes.

CALORIES BURNED: 150-180

COMMENTS

The use of inclines and declines is an important strategy to develop early in your training.

2

STAIR RUN/STEP-UPS
TOTAL TIME: 25-30 minutes

WARM-UP: Easy run for 5 minutes; 3-minute stretch.

WORKOUT

Activity: Climb a flight of stairs or the equivalent of two floors (available at local football fields and other facilities), and then return down with speed between walking and running. Rest 10 seconds before ascending a second time. Each time you climb the stairs, add an additional 5 seconds to your recovery period (for example, 10 + 5 + 5 + 5 . . .). Try to run the stairs 10 to 15 times.

Distance: Not relevant

Time: 10-12 minutes

Pace: Half-sprint

Effort: RPE 4-6; % max heart rate 70-84

COOL-DOWN: Walk halfway up the stairs, then down, then stretch for 5 minutes.

CALORIES BURNED: 150-180

COMMENTS

Stair running is great for leg development, but if stairs aren't available, use a 4- to 6-inch high bench or step instead. Using the exercise times listed for this workout, step up onto the bench and back down by alternating the lead foot every 20 step-ups; step 20 more, then use recovery periods as noted above.

WORKOUT 3

PACED SPRINTS
TOTAL TIME: 30-35 minutes

3

WARM-UP: Swim an easy crawlstroke for 5 minutes; stretch for 5 minutes.

WORKOUT

Activity: Swimming pool workout

Distances: Yards or meters

Distance	Time	Recovery
25 × 6	20-25 seconds	15 seconds
50 × 4	50-60 seconds	30 seconds
100 × 2	1:40-2:00	60 seconds

Note. Rest or recover for 2 minutes between sets.

Time: 20-25 minutes

Pace: Sprint/swim hard

Effort: RPE 4-5; % max heart rate 70-79

COOL-DOWN: Swim easy for 5 minutes and stretch.

CALORIES BURNED: 140-175

COMMENTS

Concentrating on swimming distances in specific times with specific recovery intervals is an important training technique for more advanced swim training.

WORKOUT 4

HILL-CLIMB CYCLING
TOTAL TIME: 25-30 minutes

WARM-UP: Ride on level roads for 5 minutes, increasing the speed to a half-sprint in the last 60 seconds.

WORKOUT

Activity: Using midrange gears, select a hill(s) to ride up, then coast down for 20 minutes—the more hill climbing the better.

Distance: Not relevant but may be 1,900 to 2,500 yards or meters

Time: 20 minutes

Pace: Ride as fast as you can while remaining in the saddle at all times.

Effort: RPE 4-5; % max heart rate 70-79

COOL-DOWN: Ride easy on level roads for 3 minutes; stretch as needed.

CALORIES BURNED: 220

COMMENTS

Hill riding in the saddle (remaining seated) is a valuable discipline for training the calves and quadriceps as well as being good for the lower back, so long as correct riding posture is maintained.

WORKOUT 5

FARTLEK RIDE
TOTAL TIME: 30-35 minutes

5

WARM-UP: Ride easy for 3 minutes, increase pace for 3 minutes, then back off to easy pace for 5 minutes.

WORKOUT

Activity: Following the warm-up, ride variable speeds for 15 minutes. Fartlek is an explosive output and speed activity, punctuated by sustained periods of easy to moderate effort. You can determine your explosive moments by selecting objects or landmarks in the distance and then riding hard to get to them. Once there, make a natural, nonstop transition to the easier output for a set distance or time. Construct your choices so that you ride easy twice as often as you ride hard. Ideally, sprint every 2 to 3 minutes.

Distance: Not relevant but may be 1,800 to 2,200 yards or meters

Time: 15 minutes

Pace: Alternating sprinting and easy riding

Effort: RPE 4-5; % max heart rate 70-79

COOL-DOWN: Ride easy for 3 minutes and stretch.

CALORIES BURNED: 165

COMMENTS

Fartlek riding helps you make quick biomechanical adaptations.

WORKOUT 6

6

HILL-CLIMB WALKING
TOTAL TIME: 30-35 minutes

WARM-UP: Walk in place or stride easily for 3 minutes. Do a 2-minute stretch; walk again for 5 minutes.

WORKOUT

Activity: Select a hill or hills and walk up it as fast as you can. Walk downhill fast as well. Repeat 3 to 6 times.

Distance: Not relevant to this workout

Time: 15 minutes

Pace: As fast as you can go

Effort: RPE 4-5; % max heart rate 70-79

COOL-DOWN: 5-minute stretch.

CALORIES BURNED: 150-180

COMMENTS

Hills force you to adapt your stride and arm motion, which is good for the calves and thighs.

WORKOUT 7

STAIR CLIMB/STEP-UPS
TOTAL TIME: 25-30 minutes

7

WARM-UP: Walk in place or walk easily for 5 minutes; stretch for 3 minutes.

WORKOUT

Activity: Use three flights of stairs or stadium stairs for your workout terrain. Pumping your arms and stepping at a lively pace, climb the stairs for 15 minutes and then cool down. (This may allow you to climb the three flights of stairs 4-8 times.)

Distance: Not relevant to this workout

Time: 15 minutes

Pace: Fast walk

Effort: RPE 4-6; % max heart rate 70-84

COOL-DOWN: Stretch for 3 to 5 minutes.

CALORIES BURNED: 150-180

COMMENTS

Quick stair work helps coordinate the interdependent movements of the upper and lower body while also working on coordination.

WORKOUT 8

8 AEROBICS CLASS BEHIND/IN FRONT OF THE INSTRUCTOR
TOTAL TIME: 25-35 minutes

WARM-UP: Do warm-up with class.

WORKOUT

Activity: Stand right behind or in front of the aerobics instructor to challenge yourself.

Distance: Not relevant to this workout

Time: 20 minutes

Pace: All-out in a low-impact aerobics class

Effort: RPE 4-5; % max heart rate 70-79

COOL-DOWN: After 3 minutes of walking to cool down, leave the room and do lengthy stretching.

CALORIES BURNED: 160-180

COMMENTS

Standing behind or in front of the instructor almost always boosts the level of your performance and intensity.

WORKOUT 9

SHOULDER WORKOUT WITH RESISTANCE MACHINES
TOTAL TIME: 25-30 minutes

9

WARM-UP: Ride stationary bike easily for 8 minutes or walk for 5 minutes.

WORKOUT

Activity: Use a preselected combination of 2 to 6 resistance machines, concentrating on the shoulder complex of muscles. Concentrate on negative lifts—make a slow return to the starting position after the lift. Form is essential. Do sets of 10 to 15 repetitions on each of the machines.

Distance: Not relevant to this workout

Time: 15-20 minutes

Pace: Slow, deliberate lifts

Effort: RPE 4-5; % max heart rate 70-79

COOL-DOWN: 5-minute stretch.

CALORIES BURNED: 90-120

COMMENTS

Think of shoulders as a complex of associations between numerous muscles, tendons, bones, nerves, and lubricating fluids (bursa). You should mix overall workouts in such a way that you address all muscle groups during a training cycle. (Over a series of 7-10 days you can work the upper body with resistance machines and the lower body with leg-dominated activities like running, cycling, stairclimbing, etc.)

10

CHEST WORKOUT WITH FREE WEIGHTS
TOTAL TIME: 25-35 minutes

WARM-UP: Walk for 5 minutes or ride a stationary bike for 8 minutes.

WORKOUT

Activity: Using dumbbells, do flys on an incline bench (2 sets of 15). Using dumbbells, do 2 sets of 15 repetitions of recline presses. Using a free bar, do 2 sets of 10 to 15 repetitions and a third set of 8.

Distance: Not relevant to this workout

Time: 15-25 minutes

Pace: Slow and deliberate

Effort: RPE 4-5; % max heart rate 70-79

COOL-DOWN: Bike or walk for 5 minutes.

CALORIES BURNED: 90-150

COMMENTS

You set the pace for this good conditioning workout, but you must use appropriate weights to allow high repetitions and proper form.

How Experts Might Use These Workouts

Because Purple zone workouts offer concentrated effort opportunities and are brief enough that they don't disrupt more complex maintenance routines, experts use them in the following ways:

- To accelerate the development of a specific body part or region that's out of proportion with total body symmetry. (Overdevelopment of a leg, arm, or shoulder is not uncommon in athletes who, by the nature of their sports, must concentrate effort on single limbs and their adjoining joints.)
- To tone down an overly ambitious workout on a day when the "down day demon" has stripped the exercisers of their motivation and the workout of its appeal.
- To refine stroke technique in the pool, which is an essential part of competitive swimming.
- To refine breathing transitions between cycling and running for persons training for triathlons. For example, athletes will pair a series of Purple zone cycling workouts with a series of Purple zone running workouts and then do a series of six pairs of workouts with rapid transitions between them.

While experts may creatively manipulate Purple zone workouts to meet broader competitive goals and to improve their fitness training, developing a knowledgeable approach to cross-training is goal enough for improving its overall value. In chapter 9, we'll explore the Yellow zone and how you can "amp up" the intensity and duration of your workouts.

| | | | **Summary Table** | |
| | | | **Purple Zone Workouts** | |
Workout	Description	Duration (minutes)	Distance/Time (intensity time)	Intensity (RPE/% MHR)
1	Up and downhill run	10-12	1,600-2,400 yards	4-6/70-84
2	Stair run/step-ups	10-12	10-15 stairclimbs	4-6/70-84
3	Paced sprints	20-25	Variable distances	4-5/70-79
4	Hill-climb cycling	20	1,900-2,500 yards	4-5/70-79
5	Fartlek ride	15	1,800-2,200 yards	4-5/70-79
6	Hill-climb walking	15	3-6 hills	4-5/70-79
7	Stair climb/ step-ups	15	4-8 climbs	4-6/70-84
8	Aerobics class behind/in front of the instructor	20	Low-impact aerobics	4-5/70-79
9	Shoulder workout with resistance machines	15-20	10-15 repetitions × 2	4-5/70-79
10	Chest workout with free weights	15-25	15 reps × 2 × 3 exercises; 8 × 1 (3rd set, 3rd exercise)	4-5/70-79

Yellow Zone

Yellow zone workouts begin to test your level of fitness within the undertaken activity. Training heart rates that approach 79% of your maximum heart rate and are maintained for 30 to 45 minutes are an encouraging measure of fitness. Yellow zone workouts at this level several times a week will produce significant cardiovascular benefits.

With cross-training, getting in three or four Yellow zone workouts during the week may well involve a blending of exercise mediums to fulfill a cardiovascular-building workout goal. When planning your individualized cross-training program, make your long-term fitness or competitive goals the primary guidelines for the blending of Yellow zone workouts.

Using Yellow Zone Workouts

When working on improving a basic fitness level, yellow zone workouts offer the best "bang for your buck," because they are challenging enough to tax your body, yet reachable by most persons who've established a solid base-level of fitness and who are hungry to increase their workouts' intensity.

Use Yellow zone workouts to test your readiness for spending more of your day working out (something which most exercisers need but don't take seriously enough). Assuming even that your existing workouts are well-conceived and productive, you must spend more time working out or rewrite your workout plan to increase your level of fitness.

Yellow zone workouts are best integrated into your overall workout plan when you choose activities that you know well and will not tire of doing. As you become more proficient at other activities, you can use them as substitute Yellow zone workouts. I would not advise using Yellow zone workouts as a stepping stone to perfecting a new activity, because that frequently leads to injury and creates an aversion to exercising. For instance, a person who has run for years but rarely biked or swam would be ill-advised to pick up cycling and swimming at the Yellow zone level to hasten the learning of these two disciplines. A better alternative—one that would reduce the likelihood of injury and increase performance— would be to continue the Yellow zone running and sandwich it with Green and Blue zone swimming and cycling workouts.

WORKOUT 1

INCLINE-DECLINE RUN
TOTAL TIME: 45-50 minutes

1

WARM-UP: Jog on a level surface for 5 minutes; then a 5-minute stretch.

WORKOUT

Activity: Use an incline you can run up and down. An 800- to 1,000-yard or meter section of trail, a shoulder of a roadway, or a sloping, lawn-covered area at a park or outdoor recreation area would be ideal. Run up the hill, pause for 10 seconds, and run down. Rest for as short a time as you need, and resume running up and down the hill. Every time you ascend the hill, add 10 seconds recovery time (e.g., 10 + 10 + 10 + 10 . . .). Repeat 2 to 4 times.

Distance: Ideally, you need an 800- to 1,000-yard or meter incline that is gradual but distinct. Total distance covered could be 1-1/2 to 2 miles.

Time: 25-30 minutes

Pace: Half-sprint

Effort: RPE 4-5; % max heart rate 70-79

COOL-DOWN: Walk halfway up the hill, then down, and then stretch for 10 minutes.

CALORIES BURNED: 375-450

COMMENTS

Even at this moderate intensity, this workout will develop your leg stamina very quickly.

2 STAIR RUN/STEP-UPS
TOTAL TIME: 45 minutes to 1 hour

WARM-UP: Easy run for 5 minutes; 5-minute stretch.

WORKOUT

Activity: Aggressively climb a flight of stairs that are the equivalent of two floors (available at local football fields and other facilities), and return down with an easy step that is between a walk and a run. Rest 10 seconds before ascending a second time. Add an additional 10 seconds to your recovery period each time you climb the stairs (e.g., 10 + 10 + 10 + 10 . . .). Repeat 2 to 4 times.

Distances: Not relevant to this workout

Time: 25-30 minutes

Pace: Aggressive 3/4 sprint

Effort: RPE 4-5; % max heart rate 70-79

COOL-DOWN: Walk halfway up stairs and then back down; stretch for 5 minutes.

CALORIES BURNED: 375-450

COMMENTS

This workout is particularly appropriate for persons who play sports or do activities that require a lot of stability and abrupt off-balance, return-to-balance movements. If stairs aren't available, a 4- to 6-inch high bench or step can be used instead. If using a bench, step up onto it and back down by alternating the lead foot at 20 step-ups, step 20 more; use recovery periods as outlined in this workout.

WORKOUT 3

PACED SPRINTS
TOTAL TIME: 30-35 minutes

3

WARM-UP: Do an easy crawlstroke for 5 minutes; stretch for 5 minutes.

WORKOUT

Activity: Swimming pool workout

Distances: Yards or meters

Distance	Time	Recovery (no activity)
25 × 8	20-25 seconds	10 seconds
50 × 6	50-60 seconds	15 seconds
100 × 3	1:40-2:00	20 seconds

Note. Rest/recover for 2 minutes before beginning a new set.

Time: 35-40 minutes

Pace: Sprint/swim hard

Effort: RPE 4-5; % max heart rate 70-79

COOL-DOWN: Easy swim for 5 minutes and stretch.

CALORIES BURNED: 385-440

COMMENTS

This is necessary training for endurance swimming.

4

BABY PYRAMID SPRINT SWIM × 2
TOTAL TIME: 55 minutes to 1 hour

WARM-UP: Easy freestyle for 200 yards or meters; stretch for 5 minutes. Half-sprint swim for 50 yards or meters; stretch for 5 minutes.

WORKOUT

Activity: Recover for 10 seconds after each 25 and 50; recover for 15 seconds after each 75. Repeat the Baby Pyramid.

Distances (yards or meters): 25, 50, 75, 75, 50, 25

Time: 25-30 minutes

Pace: Sprint as fast as you can go.

Effort: 4-6 RPE; % max heart rate 70-84

COOL-DOWN: Swim an easy 200 to 300 yards or meters; stretch for 5 minutes.

CALORIES BURNED: 275-330

COMMENTS

Repeating Baby Pyramids to increase training duration is an excellent transition to longer interval pyramids.

WORKOUT 5

HILL-CLIMB CYCLING
TOTAL TIME: 40-50 minutes

5

WARM-UP: Ride on level roads for 5 minutes, and then move right into the workout by immediately challenging the hill.

WORKOUT

Activity: Using middle range gears, select a hill or hills to ride up and coast down repeatedly for 30 to 40 minutes. The more hill climbing, the better.

Distance: Not relevant to this workout

Time: 30-40 minutes

Pace: Ride as fast as you can while remaining in the saddle at all times.

Effort: RPE 4-5; % max heart rate: 70-79

COOL-DOWN: Ride easy on level roads for 5 minutes; stretch as needed.

CALORIES BURNED: 330-440

COMMENTS

Lengthening your hill rides while you remain in the saddle enhances long-distance riding ability. Multiple hill rides of 2 to 7 miles are not at all unusual components of an overall 25- to 70-mile training ride.

WORKOUT 6

FARTLEK RIDE
TOTAL TIME: 45 minutes to 1 hour

WARM-UP: On level terrain, ride 3 minutes easy, 3 moderate, and 3 intense. Do leg stretches for 3 minutes.

WORKOUT

Activity: Ride variable speeds for the 30- to 40-minute period of the workout that follows the warm-up. Select the duration of your sprint stages either by time (30-90 seconds) or by distance (from where you are to another predetermined point). Always ride easy/moderate for twice as long as you sprint. You select the number of times you increase the pace. On longer rides, longer sprints might come every 3 to 5 minutes.

Distance: Not relevant, but could be 2 to 5 miles

Time: 30-40 minutes

Pace: Alternating sprinting and easy riding

Effort: RPE 4-5; % max heart rate 70-79

COOL-DOWN: Ride easy for 5 minutes and stretch.

CALORIES BURNED: 330-440

COMMENTS

Varying the pace of exertion during workouts is a valuable addition to training for competitive running, open-water swimming, cycling, and triathlons, because changing pace often mimics race situations where you must respond to crowding, bumping, and the like.

WORKOUT 7

STAIR CLIMB/STEP-UPS

TOTAL TIME: 50 minutes to 1 hour

WARM-UP: Walk in place or walk easy for 5 minutes; stretch for 5 minutes.

WORKOUT

Activity: Use three flights of stairs or stadium stairs as your workout terrain. Pumping your arms and stepping to a lively pace, climb stairs for 10 minutes. Stretch for 3 minutes; resume climbing for two more 10-minute segments, stretching for 3 minutes between them.

Distance: Not relevant to this workout

Time: 30-40 minutes

Pace: Fast walk

Effort: RPE 4-5; % max heart rate 70-79

COOL-DOWN: Stretch for 5 minutes.

CALORIES BURNED: 350-450

COMMENTS

This is a grand endurance builder, but you need to stretch at selected intervals as noted in the workout.

WORKOUT 8

8 VIDEO AEROBICS WITH PARTNER
TOTAL TIME: 45 minutes to 1 hour

WARM-UP: Follow the videotape warm-up with a partner for 5 minutes.

WORKOUT

Activity: Use an aerobics tape, low- or high-impact, and have plenty of room for yourself and a partner to exercise.

Distance: Not relevant to this workout

Time: 40-45 minutes

Pace: In accord with the videotape and the movements of your partner

Effort: RPE 4-5; % max heart rate 70-79

COOL-DOWN: Stretch together, giving mutual assistance when appropriate.

CALORIES BURNED: 320-360

COMMENTS

Sometimes, partners add pace and intensity to a video workout; always be selective and careful when choosing workout partners.

WORKOUT 9

SHOULDER WORKOUT WITH RESISTANCE MACHINES

TOTAL TIME: 40-45 minutes

WARM-UP: Stationary bike for 8 minutes or walk for 5 minutes.

WORKOUT

Activity: Use a preselected combination of 2 to 6 resistance machines, concentrating on the shoulder complex of muscles. Focus on negative lifts—a slow return to starting position after the lift. Form is essential. Do 2 sets of 10 to 15 repetitions on each machine. After the first series with all machines, stretch for 3 to 5 minutes. Repeat in reverse order (start on the last machine first).

Distance: Not relevant to this workout

Time: 30-35 minutes

Pace: Slow, deliberate lifts

Effort: RPE 4; % max heart rate 70-74

COOL-DOWN: 5-minute stretch.

CALORIES BURNED: 180-210

COMMENTS

You can best develop shoulder strength for use in sports and in life when you complement your strength training with shoulder flexibility stretches. However, be sure to challenge your other muscle systems as well with concentrated weight training on other days and at other times.

10

CHEST WORKOUT WITH FREE WEIGHTS

TOTAL TIME: 45-50 minutes

WARM-UP: Walk for 10 minutes or ride a stationary bike for 12 minutes.

WORKOUT

Activity: Using a freebar, do high repetitions (10-15) for 3 sets. Using dumbbells, select weights that allow you to properly lift them for the exercise yet are heavy enough to make it difficult for you to do any more than 3 sets of 6 to 8 repetitions for flys and recline presses. Return to the freebar for 2 sets of 10 to 15 repetitions.

Distance: Not relevant to this workout

Time: 25-35 minutes

Pace: Slow and deliberate

Effort: RPE 4; % max heart rate 70-74

COOL-DOWN: Bike or walk for 5 minutes.

CALORIES BURNED: 150-210

COMMENTS

Developing the chest muscles is popular the world over, and to achieve the best balance, you need to vary the types of resistance exercises used to build the chest; the ones offered in this workout are only a sampling of the many that exist.

How Experts Might Use These Workouts

Experts might use the Yellow zone as precompetition "tune-up" workouts for the following reasons:

- The heart rate is raised sufficiently to allow them to perform at a high level of technical arousal without overly taxing the body's ability to perform at such a level.
- The length of the workout can easily be pared to an appropriate length relative to the length of the competition, assuming, for example, that it is longer than a 5K run, 10K bike, or short course swim.
- The athletes can get close to race pace but stay far enough below it that they do not deplete energy stores.

Experts also use Yellow zone workouts for long-distance workouts and for far-over-distance workouts, also known as "mega-length" workouts (20-plus-mile training runs, 100-mile bike rides, two-hour swims).

In the next chapter, you'll be introduced to "hot training" where the heart rate is 80% to 95% of the maximum for less than 25 minutes. Think of this new training zone (the Orange zone) as hot, because performing at this intensity charges your muscles and blood flow, creating the sensation of heat. Hot also suggests something akin to sage advice when exercising in the 80% to 95% zone: "**H**old **O**n **T**ightly!"

Workout	Description	Duration (minutes)	Distance/Time (intensity time)	Intensity (RPE/% MHR)
	Summary Table			
	Yellow Zone Workouts			
1	Incline-decline run	25-30	1–1-1/2 miles	4-5/70-79
2	Stair run/step-ups	25-30	2,000-3,000 yards or meters	4-5/70-79
3	Paced sprints	35-40	Variable distances	4-5/70-79
4	Baby Pyramid sprint swim × 2	25-30	Variable distances	4-6/70-84
5	Hill-climb cycling	30-40	Multiple climbs	4-5/70-79
6	Fartlek ride	30-40	2-5 miles	4-5/70-79
7	Stair climb/ step-ups	30-40	Three 10-minute climbs	4-5/70-79
8	Video aerobics with partner	40-45	Video aerobic tape	4-5/70-79
9	Shoulder workout with resistance machines	30-35	10-15 reps × 2-6	4/70-74
10	Chest workout with free weights	25-35	10-15 reps × 3, 6-8 reps × 3, and 10-15 reps × 2	4/70-74

10

Orange Zone

Orange zone workouts are introductions to master-level workouts (the highest performance workouts), and they give you a chance to learn how to modify an exercise session to meet your unique needs and tastes for these hot workouts.

Orange zone workouts test your willingness to push your body and your potential for competition in any of a number of venues.

Using Orange Zone Workouts

Orange zone workouts measure your ability to execute movements and routines at a higher level of intensity. During even a short duration, your heart rate may be anywhere from 80% to 95% to even 100% of your maximum heart rate for given periods.

Your selection of a training heart rate depends on the activity in which you are engaged and your reasons for choosing it. When engaging in Orange zone workouts, I recommend exercisers select only those activities they know well.

Let's say you enjoy cycling very much and that you're traveling maximum distances during fartlek rides and hill climbs. Look at Yellow zone Workouts 5 and 6, and assess the demands on your heart by trying them and checking your pulse. Do this several times and then figure your training heart rate based, in part, on your RPE.

This evaluative process will assess your training potential for cycling and if all goes well, you may want to apply it to other self-challenging workouts about which you feel confident.

When testing your ability to execute an activity at a higher level of intensity for a longer period of time, use the lower training heart rate (80%) of the Orange zone range for a maximum of 24 minutes. The more consistently satisfied you are with this level of exertion, the closer you are to making serious choices about numerous competitive opportunities.

WORKOUT 1

PACED TRACK INTERVAL WORKOUTS
TOTAL TIME: 30-35 minutes

WARM-UP: Warm up to prevent injuries to muscles and tendons. Run easy for 5 minutes, stretch for 10 minutes, run 4 half-speed, 20-yard sprints on grass, stretch, run 2 full-speed, 20-yard sprints on the grass, and finish the warm-up with a thorough stretch.

WORKOUT

Activity: Track sprint work

Distances: Yards or meters

Full-speed sprint distance	Walking recovery distance
25	50
50	100
25	50
50	200
100	300

Repeat the above 1 to 3 times if time permits.

Time: 20-25 minutes

Pace: Full-speed sprints; moderate-speed walk

Effort: RPE 6-7; % max heart rate 80-89

COOL-DOWN: Run easy for 5 minutes and thoroughly stretch.

CALORIES BURNED: 400-500

COMMENTS

Sprint intervals are important in every sport that requires explosive execution. Muscle specificity is most evident in sprint training because the demands of competitive sprinting to pass opponents or streak to the finish line cannot be learned through long-distance or endurance riding. Cyclists need sprint training to "teach" their muscles to "break away" from the pack. Start gradually and build up to the distances.

2

PULL, SWIM, KICK
TOTAL TIME: 25-35 minutes

WARM-UP: Swim an easy 300 yards or meters; stretch for 3 minutes.

WORKOUT

Activity: First swim with a pull buoy (no kick), release the buoy and, without stopping, begin swimming (with kick) for a set distance. Finally, swim using a kickboard and kick only for a set distance.

Distances: Yards or meters

Sets you pull (P), swim (S), and kick (K)	Recovery* between sets
25 (25-P, 25-S, 25-K)	60 seconds
50 (50-P, 50-S, 50-K)	1:30
75 (75-P, 75-S, 75-K)	1:30
100 (100-P, 100-S, 100-K)	Cool-down

*Complete inactivity

Time: 15-20 minutes

Pace: At your pace; mark your times for comparison with future workouts.

Effort: RPE 7-8; % max heart rate 85-95

COOL-DOWN: Swim an easy 200 yards or meters; stretch.

CALORIES BURNED: 210-280+

COMMENTS

You never really use a pull-swim-kick routine in competition, but the challenge it poses for you to adapt and maintain pace is appropriate to overall cross-training and also provides variety in a training schedule.

WORKOUT 3

PYRAMID SWIM
TOTAL TIME: 25-30 minutes

3

WARM-UP: Swim at moderate pace for 200 yards or meters; 5-minute stretch.

WORKOUT

Activity: Swimming pool workout

Distances: Yards or meters

Distance	Recovery* between sets
25	10 seconds
50	15 seconds
75	20 seconds
100	30 seconds
100	45 seconds
75	30 seconds
50	20 seconds
25	Cool-down

*Complete inactivity

Time: 15-20 minutes

Pace: Full speed

Effort: RPE 6-8; % max heart rate 80-95

COOL-DOWN: Swim an easy 200 yards or meters and stretch.

CALORIES BURNED: 210-350+

COMMENTS

Swimming increasingly longer distances with predetermined recovery times is excellent both physiologically and psychologically. As a training and competitive medium, water often defeats the athlete, but this kind of workout helps to develop your confidence when in the water.

WORKOUT 4

4

TIMED-INTERVAL RIDE
TOTAL TIME: 30-40 minutes

WARM-UP: Ride at moderate pace for 5 minutes.

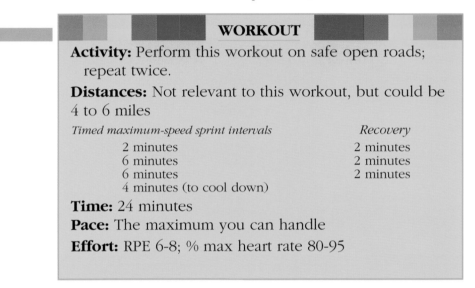

WORKOUT

Activity: Perform this workout on safe open roads; repeat twice.

Distances: Not relevant to this workout, but could be 4 to 6 miles

Timed maximum-speed sprint intervals	Recovery
2 minutes	2 minutes
6 minutes	2 minutes
6 minutes	2 minutes
4 minutes (to cool down)	

Time: 24 minutes

Pace: The maximum you can handle

Effort: RPE 6-8; % max heart rate 80-95

COOL-DOWN: Ride easy for 5 minutes; stretch.

CALORIES BURNED: 336+

COMMENTS

Timed-interval riding offers a disciplined training technique that is useful for conditioning your body to make transitions.

WORKOUT 5

DISTANCE RIDE
TOTAL TIME: 25-30 minutes

5

WARM-UP: Stand in place and do toe and heel raises for 1 minute; pause for 30 seconds and repeat the process. Ride moderately for 3 to 5 minutes.

WORKOUT

Activity: You can approach this as a time-trial ride by establishing a set riding time and measuring the distance traveled by speedometer or by a landmark against which you can compare future rides.

Distance: You determine, based on pedal speed (approximately 5-10 miles).

Time: 20 minutes

Pace: 15-25+ miles per hour

Effort: RPE 6-8; % max heart rate 80-95

COOL-DOWN: Ride easy for 5 minutes; stretch.

CALORIES BURNED: 210+

COMMENTS

At this upper level of training, establishing baseline values for measuring progress is a critical strategy for competitive athletes and serious cross-trainers.

WORKOUT 6

PACED TRACK INTERVALS (WALKING)

TOTAL TIME: 20-25 minutes

WARM-UP: Walk twice around the track; stretch for 5 minutes.

WORKOUT

Activity: Very brisk walking on a measured track or measured walking surface

Distances: Yards or meters

Interval × repetitions	Recovery
50 × 4	100
100 × 2	300

Time: 10-15 minutes; do intervals only once.

Pace: As fast as you can without jogging for the intervals; moderate during recovery

Effort: RPE 6-7; % max heart rate 80-89

COOL-DOWN: Walk moderately for 5 minutes; stretch.

CALORIES BURNED: 140-210+

COMMENTS

Fast-paced walking is an art and a sport, and you can use this workout as a filler for those times you feel your body needs a quick, low-impact "punch."

WORKOUT 7

VIDEO AEROBICS WITH PARTNER
TOTAL TIME: 20-30 minutes

WARM-UP: Do the warm-up as indicated on the tape.

WORKOUT

Activity: At-home video workout

Distance: Not relevant to this workout

Time: 20-30 minutes

Pace: Maximum performance to an advanced aerobic training videotape, with vocalizations from you and your partner—yells and hoots, along with participatory and encouraging language—to play along with the instructor

Effort: RPE 5-7; % max heart rate 80-89

COOL-DOWN: Walk in place for 3 to 5 minutes; stretch with the tape after fast-forwarding tape to flexibility portion, or stretch on your own with your partner.

CALORIES BURNED: 240+

COMMENTS

Because the quality of tapes and workouts are quite variable, you've got to preview all aerobics tapes and identify those most appropriate for your training needs.

WORKOUT 8

8

STEP AEROBICS
TOTAL TIME: 30-35 minutes

WARM-UP: Warm up in a step aerobics class.

WORKOUT

Activity: Step aerobics class

Distance: Not relevant to this workout

Time: 20 minutes

Pace: Maximum performance with concentration on form and execution

Effort: RPE 5-7; % max heart rate 80-89

COOL-DOWN: Leave the class and walk in place, ride a stationary bike, or use a stairclimber at a very low level for 3 to 5 minutes.

CALORIES BURNED: 240

COMMENTS

Think of step aerobics as a complementary workout to your overall sports training.

WORKOUT 9

CHEST OR BACK BLASTS
TOTAL TIME: 20-30 minutes

WARM-UP: Bike, walk, or stairclimb for 5 to 10 minutes.

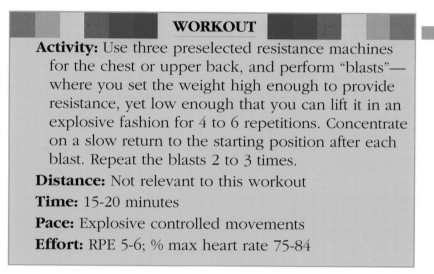

WORKOUT

Activity: Use three preselected resistance machines for the chest or upper back, and perform "blasts"— where you set the weight high enough to provide resistance, yet low enough that you can lift it in an explosive fashion for 4 to 6 repetitions. Concentrate on a slow return to the starting position after each blast. Repeat the blasts 2 to 3 times.

Distance: Not relevant to this workout

Time: 15-20 minutes

Pace: Explosive controlled movements

Effort: RPE 5-6; % max heart rate 75-84

COOL-DOWN: Bike, walk, or stair climb for 5 to 10 minutes.

CALORIES BURNED: 135-180

COMMENTS

Blasts are a method of "flexing" your strength and serve as an occasional alternative to use for maintaining strength.

10

ABDOMINAL RESISTANCE WORK

TOTAL TIME: 20-25 minutes

WARM-UP: Walk in place for 3 minutes; shake out and begin the workout.

WORKOUT

Activity: Using a prerecorded 15- to 20-minute tape of your favorite music, lie on your back on an exercise mat and begin performing abdominal resistance exercises as soon as the tape begins. Exercise your abdominals continuously until the tape stops. If you are thoughtful in your selection of music, you can create variations in the resistance exercises you use to work the abdominals.

Distance: Not relevant to this workout

Time: 15-20 minutes

Pace: Maximum performance; you can determine the pace by the music you select and thus exercise to many different paces during the workout.

Effort: 5-6 RPE; % max heart rate 75-84

COOL-DOWN: Do lower back arches, spinal stretches, and hip stretches.

CALORIES BURNED: 135-180

COMMENTS

You should have already developed a repertoire of abdominal exercises to use before trying this workout. Learning to do abdominal work to music for a continuous period accelerates the development of abdominal stamina—an essential ingredient in protecting the lower back during vigorous workouts or competitions.

How Experts Might Use These Workouts

Orange zone workouts are not "no pain, no gain" endeavors, but no workout should project working through pain as the primary goal. Expert competitors have learned how to take advantage of the inevitable pain in competition by learning to work *with* it and not through it and to work in response to it, making on-the-spot adaptations in form, style, technique, or in other elements of their execution. For experts, Orange zone workouts may be planned to provide

- an opportunity to work with pain;
- an intense but short, final tune-up before racing; and
- a strategy for middle-distance runners and sprinters, short-course swimmers, aerobic competitors, race walkers, and for hill climbers in cycling.

Experts use a high training heart rate during the emulation of competition to reinforce expected gains in ability and sometimes to refine minor technical adjustments, such as hand position, race-pace strategy, or warm-up routines.

In the next chapter, you'll encounter the fullest challenge of the colored zone training model in this book and be invited to investigate a host of multiactivity Red zone workouts. So, get going with your Orange zone workouts!

| | | | Summary Table | |
| | | | Orange Zone Workouts | |
Workout	Description	Duration (minutes)	Distance/Time (intensity time)	Intensity (RPE/% MHR)
1	Paced track interval workouts	20-25	Variable distances	6-7/80-89
2	Pull, swim, kick	15-20	Variable distances, full speed	7-8/85-95
3	Pyramid swim	15-20	Variable distances, full speed	6-8/80-95
4	Timed-interval ride	24	4-6 miles	6-8/80-95
5	Distance ride	20	5-10 miles	6-8/80-95
6	Paced track intervals (walking)	10-15	Variable distances	6-7/80-89
7	Video aerobics with partner	20-30	Video aerobic tape	5-7/80-89
8	Step aerobics	20	Step aerobics class	5-7/80-89
9	Chest or back blasts	15-20	3 resistance machines × 2-3	5-6/75-84
10	Abdominal resistance work	15-20	Floorwork	5-6/75-84

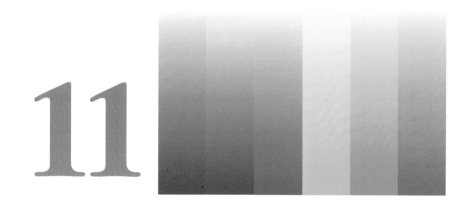

Red Zone

If the Orange zone was hot, then the Red zone is sizzling! I don't consider the Red zone accessible to all exercisers; more to the point, it's actually inhospitable to all but the trained and seasoned. Red zone workouts connote a heart rate 80% to 95% of maximum, maintained for over 25 minutes.

The challenge with Red zone workouts is maintaining pace, form, muscle function, and focus on the exercise/activity. Without a substantial fitness base, which includes a high-carbohydrate, very low-fat diet that provides only high-quality protein, a body composition that's low in fat and high in lean mass, and deliberately planned rest days appropriate to a competitive training schedule, Red zone workouts are fruitless and potentially injurious. On the other hand, given the required fitness base, Red zone workouts are the Ferraris of fitness training.

Using Red Zone Workouts

As suggested previously, only well-trained and fit individuals should include Red zone workouts in their training plans. For these persons, Red zone workouts will most frequently provide significant fitness and performance boosts.

The idea of working anywhere over 90% of maximum heart rate has been called a number of things, all of which suggest the same thing—

improvement or high performance. "Boosters" are Red zone workouts intended to improve a race time. "Redlining" is a form of Red zone workout done at a very high training heart rate on a scheduled basis during the week. "Hot laps," "hot ladders," and "hot ropes" all describe versions of Red zone workouts, and all are designed for the fit exerciser and competitive athlete.

The workouts that follow should not be used without appropriate preparation. If you think it better to sample them beforehand, you may use these workouts at a lower level of intensity and for variable time periods.

WORKOUT 1

PACED-TRACK-INTERVAL SPRINTS
TOTAL TIME: 1 hour to 1 hour 10 minutes

1

WARM-UP: Run easy for 5 minutes (2-3 laps around the track), stretch for 10 minutes, run 4 half-speed, 20-yard sprints on grass; stretch. Run 2 full-speed, 20-yard sprints on the grass; stretch.

WORKOUT

Activity: Interval sprints on a regulation track

Distances: Yards or meters

Full-speed sprint distances × reps	Walk/jog recovery distance
25 × 2	50
50 × 3	100
100 × 2	300
50 × 6	150

Repeat 2 to 5 times as long as you continue to turn in times similar to your earlier sprints. If your performance is waning and earlier times seem impossible to attain, refocus your workout and work at achieving consistency in your effort relative to each set of intervals.

Time: 40 minutes

Pace: Full-speed sprints; moderate-speed walk/jog

Effort: RPE 8-10; % max heart rate 90-100

COOL-DOWN: Run easy for 5 minutes and stretch for 10 minutes.

CALORIES BURNED: 800

COMMENTS

Sprint workouts aren't for everyone and should not be attempted without a history of explosive running. The concept of training near maximum levels of exertion, known as "redlining," is advised for only short duration workouts. Sprint intervals (recovery periods) are not redline workouts.

WORKOUT 2

2

DISTANCE RUN
TOTAL TIME: 40-50 minutes

WARM-UP: Begin distance runs with 3 to 5 minutes of easy running, building into your training speed, or run easy for 3 to 5 minutes and stretch before beginning your training run.

WORKOUT

Activity: Running on a track or safe open roads

Distance: 5 miles minimum; 7 miles maximum

Time: 30-40 minutes

Pace: 6-minute mile pace

Effort: RPE 8-10; % max heart rate 90-100

COOL-DOWN: Walk on level terrain for 5 minutes; walk backwards for 3 minutes, making sure to touch your heels to the ground; stretch.

CALORIES BURNED: 600-800

COMMENTS

Distance runs are habit forming, and it's important from a cross-training perspective to use distance runs selectively as complementary workout activities.

WORKOUT 3

PULL, SWIM, KICK
TOTAL TIME: 45 minutes to 1 hour

3

WARM-UP: Swim an easy 300 yards or meters; stretch for 3 minutes.

WORKOUT

Activity: Pool swimming

Distances: Yards or meters

Sets you swim (S), pull (P), and kick (K)	Recovery between sets
25-P, 25-S, 25-K × 3	60 seconds
50-P, 50-S, 50-K × 3	1:30
75-P, 75-S, 75-K × 2	1:30
100-P, 100-S, 100-K × 2	2:00; Cool-down

Time: 25-40 minutes

Pace: Full speed; check your times and improve them with each subsequent P-S-K workout.

Effort: RPE 8-10; % max heart rate 90-100

COOL-DOWN: Swim an easy 200 yards or meters; stretch.

CALORIES BURNED: 350-560

COMMENTS

Pull-swim-kick workouts have a place in everyone's precompetition cross-training program.

WORKOUT 4

PYRAMID SWIM
TOTAL TIME: 45 minutes to 1 hour

WARM-UP: Swim at a moderate pace for 500 yards or meters; 5-minute stretch.

WORKOUT

Activity: Pool swimming

Distances: Yards or meters

Distance	Recovery between sets
Twice at each distance	1st set/2nd set
25	5/10 seconds
50	5/10 seconds
75	10/20 seconds
100	10/20 seconds
100	20/40 seconds
75	10/20 seconds
50	5/10 seconds
25	2:00/cool-down

Time: 25-30 minutes

Pace: Full speed

Effort: RPE 8-10; % max heart rate 90-100

COOL-DOWN: Swim an easy 200 yards or meters and stretch.

CALORIES BURNED: 350-420

COMMENTS

These are the kinds of swim workouts that add zest (and fatigue), both physiologically and psychologically, to one's training. This kind of workout helps develop confidence in the water. To add variety to the challenge of this workout, you may alter the strokes used when descending the pyramid.

WORKOUT 5

TIMED-INTERVAL RIDE

TOTAL TIME: 1 hour to 1 hour 10 minutes

WARM-UP: Ride at a moderate pace for 5 minutes.

WORKOUT

Activity: Use an open road with little traffic or an indoor trainer or exercise cycle.

Distance: Not relevant to this workout

Time: 50 minutes

Timed maximum-speed sprint intervals	Recovery
5 minutes	2 minutes
8 minutes	4 minutes
15 minutes	6 minutes
8 minutes	Cool-down

Pace: The maximum you can handle

Effort: RPE 8-10; % max heart rate 90-100

COOL-DOWN: Ride easy for 5 minutes; stretch.

CALORIES BURNED: 700

COMMENTS

This is an endurance and stamina-building workout.

WORKOUT 6

6

DISTANCE RIDE

TOTAL TIME: 50 minutes to 1 hour 10 minutes

WARM-UP: Stand in place and do toe and heel raises for 2 minutes. Ride moderately for 3 to 5 minutes.

WORKOUT

Activity: Approach this as a timed ride for distance by riding for a set time (e.g., 40 minutes), and then measuring the distance traveled by speedometer or by a landmark against which you can compare future rides.

Distance: You determine, based on pedal speed (approximately 10-16 miles).

Time: 40 minutes

Pace: 15-25 miles per hour

Effort: RPE 8-10; % max heart rate 90-100

COOL-DOWN: Ride easy for 5 minutes; stretch.

CALORIES BURNED: 560

COMMENTS

Depending on your training needs, these longer rides are a fine transition for the 20- to 50-mile training rides.

WORKOUT 7

DISTANCE WALK
TOTAL TIME: 1 hour

7

WARM-UP: Begin with a 3-minute easy pace, and move right into the workout.

WORKOUT

Activity: Use a measured distance of open road or track.

Distance: 4 miles

Time: 50 minutes

Pace: 12-minute mile pace

Effort: RPE 6-8; % max heart rate 80-95

COOL-DOWN: Walk for 3 to 5 minutes and stretch.

CALORIES BURNED: 750

COMMENTS

Like cycling, baseline comparisons of distances covered in specific timed intervals can be used to measure improvement as training hours add up. These are great workouts for persons in training for competition and for those who want to put in the exercise time but can't run, cycle, swim, or do aerobics.

8

STEP AEROBICS CLASS

TOTAL TIME: 1 hour to 1 hour 30 minutes

WARM-UP: Warm up in a step aerobics class.

WORKOUT

Activity: Attend a step aerobics workout in a local fitness facility (could also be done at home with a video and the proper equipment).

Distance: Not relevant to this workout

Time: 1 hour to 1 hour 30 minutes

Pace: Maximum performance with concentration on form and execution

Effort: RPE 7-10; % max heart rate 85-100

COOL-DOWN: Do as instructed in class.

CALORIES BURNED: 600-900

COMMENTS

Done correctly, step aerobics can be an interesting and productive addition to your overall training.

WORKOUT 9

CHEST AND BACK BLASTS
TOTAL TIME: 55 minutes to 1 hour

9

WARM-UP: Bike, walk, or stair climb for 10 minutes; 3- to 5-minute upper body stretch.

WORKOUT

Activity: Use preselected resistance machines for the upper back and free-weight exercises for the chest. Perform blasts first on the back, then the chest, alternating throughout the workout. Be sure to set the weight high enough to provide resistance yet low enough so you can lift it in an explosive fashion for 4 to 6 repetitions. Concentrate on a slow return to the starting position after each of the blasts. Do the blasts for 30 to 35 minutes.

Distance: Not relevant to this workout

Time: 30-35 minutes

Pace: Explosive controlled movements

Effort: RPE 5-6; % max heart rate 75-84

COOL-DOWN: Bike, walk, or stair climb for 5 to 10 minutes; stretch.

CALORIES BURNED: 270-315

COMMENTS

To concentrate on negative lifts with free weights, you must use a poundage that is relatively easy to lift (50%-60% of a maximum lift). These values should be determined before beginning this and similar workouts.

10

ABDOMINAL RESISTANCE WORK

TOTAL TIME: 45 minutes

WARM-UP: Cycle, jog, run, walk, stairclimb for 10 minutes.

WORKOUT

Activity: Using weight room apparatus and/or abdominal machines, do the following:

Exercise	Sets/repetitions	Recovery between sets
Cable pull-downs	3/12, 10, 8	60 seconds
Legs on bench crunches	3/20+	60 seconds
Incline crunches	3/20+	60 seconds

Note. Allow 2-minute transitions between exercises. Repeat as many times as desired.

Distance: Not relevant to this workout

Time: 35 minutes

Pace: Maximum performance; you determine by the exercises you select.

Effort: RPE 5-6; % max heart rate 75-84

COOL-DOWN: Do lower back arches, spinal stretches, hip stretches, and upper body stretches.

CALORIES BURNED: 315

COMMENTS

Abdominal strength can be easily developed, because you can work your abdominal muscles repeatedly with little risk of failure. Incorporate a variety of approaches to strengthening all four muscle groups of the abdominals. Select weights that permit you to perform the exercise without straining (which leads to injury in other parts of the body).

How Experts Might Use These Workouts

Just as Orange zone workouts may be used as tune-ups for racing, Red zone workouts may be used to

- simulate race intensity during training,
- mimic performance demand as experts would do in the case of aerobics and weight training, and
- provide high-level training during the intervals between scheduled competitions.

Very-high-level trainers and competitors vary the duration of Red zone workouts as a matter of course during the week from the minimum of at least 30 minutes each time to as much as 60 to 90 minutes on a nonrace day. Used correctly, Red zone workouts are highly productive; used incorrectly, they may lead to injury.

Next, we'll look at the final section of the book, and put it all together. Part III will provide an opportunity for you to become a cross-trainer, a multisport athlete, or a pleasantly versatile exerciser. It's now up to you, so choose wisely!

Workout	Description	Duration (minutes)	Distance/time (intensity time)	Intensity (RPE/% MHR)
		Summary Table		
		Red Zone Workouts		
1	Paced-track-interval sprints	40	Variable distances	8-10/90-100
2	Distance run	30-40	5-7 miles	8-10/90-100
3	Pull, swim, kick	25-40	Variable distances, full speed	8-10/90-100
4	Pyramid swim	25-30	Variable distances, full speed	8-10/90-100
5	Timed-interval ride	50	Full speed	8-10/90-100
6	Distance ride	40	10-16 miles	8-10/90-100
7	Distance walk	50	4 miles	6-8/80-95
8	Step aerobics class	1 hour to 1 hour 30 minutes	Class at fitness club	7-10/85-100
9	Chest and back blasts	30-35	4-6 repetitions × 5	5-6/75-84
10	Abdominal resistance work	35	Free machines & freebars/apparatus × 2-3	5-6/75-84

PART III

TRAINING BY THE WORKOUT ZONES

Now that you understand the parameters of the workout zones, you're ready to take advantage of this knowledge and develop a cross-training program targeting your fitness needs and interests.

If you aspire to become a triathlete or a multisport competitor, to train for single-sport competitive athletics, to improve your performance in recreational sports, to become very fit, or to ensure variety in your overall workout routine (frequent or not), the following chapters will help you construct the workout program you need.

The color-coded workout zones are a training aid to guide you in selecting workouts appropriate to your fitness level, not necessarily a graduation ladder that you must ascend to earn the right to perform higher intensity workouts. You may, however, find this approach an attractive option. A novice exerciser might construct a cross-training program from primarily Green, Blue, and Purple zones; a recreational sports enthusiast might choose from primarily Purple, Yellow, and perhaps Orange zone workouts; and a triathlete would use primarily Orange and Red zone workouts, with appropriate visitation to other zones during precompetition tapering, while injured, or for a training holiday.

It's important to remember that workout zones are fluid, and depending on one's need, any exerciser or superathlete can select any color zone. Each of the preceding chapters on workout zones has included a section at the end discussing how expert trainers might use different workouts.

Although the scope of workouts has addressed only six exercise activities, the model for combining activities presented here is applicable to the full range. Chapter 12 teaches you how to set up a cross-training program, and chapter 13 explains and provides samples of multiactivity workouts. Chapter 14 offers you a variety of objective and subjective measures to chart your progress with cross-training.

12

Setting Up Your Own Program

The heart and soul of a productive and highly satisfying cross-training program is the tactical framework, upon which it is built, and when you approach training with a tactical framework you can take any one of the basic programs in this chapter and reshape it into one that's right for your cross-training fitness needs. I characterize this tactical framework as the **APPEAL** of cross-training.

APPEAL of Cross-Training

1. Anticipatory **A**ttitude. Be psyched up for your workouts, just as you would be for competition!
2. Purposeful **P**lanning. Make each workout an important step toward helping you achieve your training goals!
3. **P**reparation, not Procrastination. Develop your skills with the necessary and basic fitness foundation.
4. **E**xecution Excellence. Don't just practice; make perfect practice.
   - Honest appraisal. Consider the demands of an activity and honestly appraise your ability to perform it.
   - Possession of native and learned skills. Do you possess the appropriate skills needed for the activity?

- Psychological commitment. Think of practice as one of the many steps toward achieving a goal. Not every workout must be a gold medal performance.
- Reliable feedback. The better the positive feedback, the greater the potential for gain.

5. **A**dventure and Atmosphere. Create safe, productive, and fun training regimens that vary your effort, your activities, and your scheduled periods of rest. Consider training partners (see Table 12.1).

6. **L**aughter and Logistics. Take your workouts seriously, but don't take yourself too seriously.

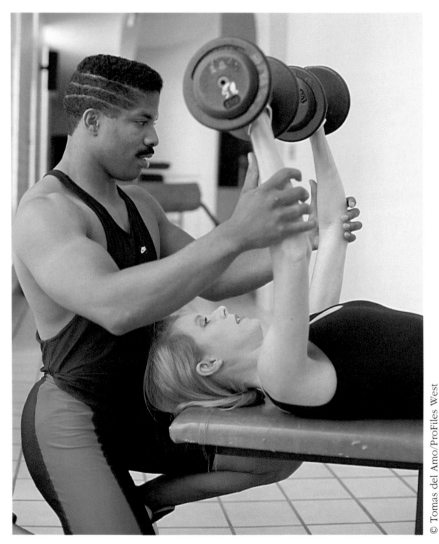

© Tomas del Amo/ProFiles West

A knowledgeable partner can be a good training aid.

| Table 12.1 |
| Training Partners—Yes or No? |

When training partners are a complement	**When training partners are a negative addiction**
When they push you to safe, yet challenging extremes	When you need your training partner to get psyched up
When you can learn anything from them—skills, attitude, training tips, nutrition, injury rehab	When your partner doesn't show up and you don't train
When you can serve as temporary mentor (helps in your application of skills)	When you give in most of the time to your partner's interests
When the partnership creates an upbeat training environment	When you rarely assert yourself and express your training needs to your partner
When you feel stuck and need a new tactic for skill development	When you pace your training on what's expected of you, rather than on reaching your potential when it's apparent you're not
When your partner challenges you to break free of a routine that may be too comfortable and not as progressive as you need to achieve your goals	When you intentionally pace down (at a time you're primed to excel) to a partner's level of training

Setting Up a One-Month Cross-Training Program

The basic concepts for setting up a program on your own are these: (a) Insist on variety; (b) don't intensely work the same muscles with weights or activity the same way day after day (or more than 2 days in a row at the upper fitness levels); (c) exercise specific muscles and muscle systems "hard," then easy, then hard or moderate over a 2- to 3-day period; (d) give areas of the body exercised in the morning an opportunity to recover while another area of the body is worked in the evening or the next morning; (e) as your training expertise increases and you progress toward more taxing workouts, use lower intensity workouts for "recovery" in the evening or next day.

Beginning/Easy

Because the emphasis of this book is developing a cross-training approach to fitness, even the novice exerciser will get to exercise as a more experienced cross-trainer would—with a.m. and p.m. workouts—but at a beginner's level of intensity and duration, with 2 full days of rest during the early weeks of the program.

With respect to expanding the 2-week program, it's best not to lengthen the duration or increase the intensity of the workouts until you are able to comfortably complete all listed workouts. Alternatively, you may choose to exercise once a day, as most exercisers do, and you may select only the morning or only the evening workouts.

Week 1

	M	Tu	W	Th	F	Sa	Su
MORNING WORKOUT	1	4		4	7	5	
EVENING WORKOUT	9	10		10	9	10	

Week 2

	M	Tu	W	Th	F	Sa	Su
MORNING WORKOUT	6	4		3	7	5	
EVENING WORKOUT	1	10		10	10	10	

Week 3

	M	Tu	W	Th	F	Sa	Su
MORNING WORKOUT	2	3	5	3	6	3	
EVENING WORKOUT	6	10	8	10	8	10	

Week 4

	M	Tu	W	Th	F	Sa	Su
MORNING WORKOUT	1	3	6	3	8	4	
EVENING WORKOUT	5	9	8	9	6	9	

Frequent/Moderate

This person has had a variety of fitness experiences but has not really engaged in organized cross-training. The habit of frequent exercise makes this person an ideal candidate for an appropriately challenging program. Again, like in the *beginning/easy* program, it's best not to lengthen the duration or increase the intensity of the workouts until you're able to comfortably complete all listed workouts. And you may use only the series of morning workouts or of evening workouts if you choose to exercise once a day.

Week 1	M	Tu	W	Th	F	Sa	Su
MORNING WORKOUT	2	3	7	3	2	4	
EVENING WORKOUT	5	10	6	10	6	9	

Week 2	M	Tu	W	Th	F	Sa	Su
MORNING WORKOUT	1	3	8	3	5	4	
EVENING WORKOUT	6	9	10	9	10	9	

Week 3	M	Tu	W	Th	F	Sa	Su
MORNING WORKOUT	1	2	6	2	5	3	
EVENING WORKOUT	6	9	10	9	10	9	

Week 4	M	Tu	W	Th	F	Sa	Su
MORNING WORKOUT	2	4	5	3	6	4,9,10	2
EVENING WORKOUT	6	9/10	1	9/10	8		

Competitive/Intense

This person requires more finely-tuned workouts and often uses cross-training to prepare for competition, or during the off-season, to build a better base or foundation for future competitive seasons. The following model programs are meant to be done twice a day as scheduled. It's common for competitive athletes' training programs to include as many as three highly specialized workouts a day, one or more of which are multiactivity workouts.

The following 2 weeks represent the general nature of workouts used by serious exercisers. These workouts, as designed, can be repeated for an extended period with new progressions brought into the plan to develop one's skills in a new sport or activity.

The following 2 weeks are precompetition weeks and do not cite specific workouts; rather, color zones are given to depict the intensity and duration of training used in preparing for competition (assuming, of course, that the athlete/exerciser has already established a foundation of exercise and fitness).

Specific workouts that are geared to the demands of the competition are generally not as varied as those used during the building of one's foundation of exercise and fitness. You'll notice that there are high-intensity, long-duration workouts occurring back to back; the activities competitors select are not intended to challenge the same muscle groups back to back but rather to enhance overall strength, stamina, and cardiovascular fitness while mentally toughening the competitive spirit.

Week 1	M	Tu	W	Th	F	Sa	Su
MORNING WORKOUT							
EVENING WORKOUT							

Week 2	M	Tu	W	Th	F	Sa	Su
MORNING WORKOUT						RACE DAY	RECOVERY
EVENING WORKOUT							

Basics to Planning a 12-Month Cross-Training Program

Although the logistics and terminology vary in different countries, *periodization* is a training concept first popularized by the Soviets and other formerly Eastern bloc countries. While such training concepts as periodization, training cycles, and zonal blocks represent a calendar-based framework in which to plan a sport or fitness training regimen, it's heartening to know that a cross-training program is at the heart of all of these.

The suggested durations for the four stages of the classic 12-month periodization are as follows:

- Preparatory period (off-season): 1-4 months
- Skills-refinement period (preseason): 1-4 months
- Competition (season): 2-4 months
- Transition (postseason): 30-45 days

Cross-Training Works!

Whatever terminology you use, the principles of generalized fitness, skill refinement, competition, and recovery or recuperation are sound ones upon which to build a 12-month cross-training program. You do not have to achieve peak performance at competition for these phases to work for you; peaking at your highest level of execution—your best bike ride, longest or fastest run, swim or walk, and so forth—is a sufficient achievement from which to recover and play with other fitness activities before you begin a new training phase.

By learning how to use this type of training strategy, you ensure more benefit and less injury from your chosen exercises and sports play. Even more important, you learn to develop a cross-training program that has an end in sight—your competition or performance high. This training strategy allows you to play with sports and activities for several weeks following competition while maintaining your fitness and your interest in creating a new cross-training adventure based on a developmental model like that of periodization.

Your Cross-Training Plan

If you're interested in an all-around fitness plan for the year, use the following Plan A. If you're looking at a competition 6 to 8 months away and you are interested in competing, use Plan B.

Plan A.   Select an appropriate sample cross-training plan from this chapter and follow it for 1 to 2 months, charting your progress and monitoring how you feel about your program.

Make appropriate modifications in your regimen, and map out a 2-month plan of activity according to the phases of periodization presented earlier (this plan can also be modified, or it can be the phases of another developmental training plan).

Overall, use these 2 to 3 months (it could just as well be 4-5 months if you've just begun an exercise routine) to develop a foundation of general fitness. Use primarily Green, Blue, and Purple zone workouts during this phase with a lot of variety.

If you are feeling and looking successful, try planning your own cross-training program to achieve a defined fitness goal by a certain time period—a month, for example.

Conspicuous and diligent record keeping and progress reports on your workouts are important ongoing elements to achieving success.

Plan to test yourself with exercise performance at monthly intervals leading up to your target date. If progress is slower than anticipated, consider modifying your training by adding two-a-day workouts, increasing intensity or duration, or changing activities. If injuries are a problem, check equipment, exercise habits, form, intensity, duration, rest or recovery patterns, and make appropriate modifications, even if it means stopping all impact activity for 2 to 4 weeks or working only in water or with elastic/rubber band resistance.

Plan B.   Select an appropriate sample cross-training plan from this chapter and follow it for 1 to 2 months, charting your progress and monitoring how you feel about your program.

Make appropriate modifications in your regimen, and map out a 4-month plan of activity according to the phases of periodization presented previously (this plan can also be modified, or it can be the phase of another developmental training plan).

Allow at least 1 to 2 months to round out your fitness foundation. Use primarily Purple, Yellow, and Orange zone workouts during this phase with a lot of variety.

Depending on skill level, use another 1 to 2 months to hone the skills necessary to compete. Use Blue and Purple zone workouts to perfect skills in the first month of training, and in the final month before competition, use Orange and Red zone workouts, tapering down for the final two weeks before competition, as illustrated earlier in the chapter.

Compete with vigor and take note of your success, but pay attention to those areas of execution that need improvement. Plan a 2- to 4-week "playtime" after competition; don't go out and try to immediately correct any deficiencies. It takes much longer to recognize your deficiencies than it does to correct them.

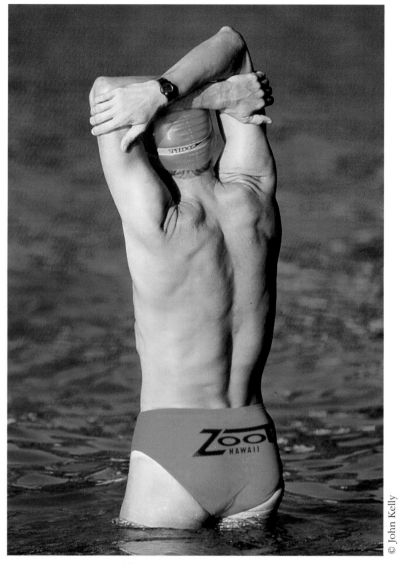

© John Kelly

Make appropriate modifications in your training so you have time to hone your skills for competition.

With Plans A or B, the bottom line is to have fun and enjoy the achievement you can attain with careful planning. Certainly, as competitions increase the demand for better technique, you will likely need coaching and specific training assistance. But if you're just getting started with cross-training at any level, you'll become your own expert planner in no time by following the guidelines in this chapter.

13

Multiple-Activity Workouts

Until now, the focus has been on incorporating variety into your overall workout program by purposefully mixing different types of workouts. Once you have perfected this cross-training routine, next you'll need to incorporate two or more different activities into the same single workout. Ultimately, you'll need to make this multiactivity workout one among many in the spectrum of workouts in your overall cross-training program. (For an example of a multiactivity workout, see chapter 12, page 137— Saturday morning's swim and weight training workout.)

For beginning exercisers as well as single-activity, frequent exercisers, multiactivity workouts add variety to training. Given the occasional need for levity, even the addition of a few rounds of horseshoes to complement or replace a planned upper-body weight workout is perfectly acceptable.

Think about it; there is nothing lost in the big picture of fitness training when a new or even a veteran exerciser opts to pitch horseshoes instead of training with dumbbells every so often. Such diversions are more important to overall exercise adherence for new and even moderate-level

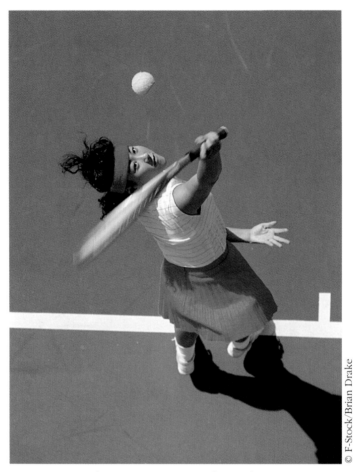

© F-Stock/Brian Drake

Any activity can be an appropriate workout when you cross-train.

exercisers than any measure of feeling that one must strictly adhere to a weight training routine or be a failure.

For more seasoned and conditioned athletes, training errors are more of an issue than adherence, because at higher levels of fitness there's actually more leeway in training breaks. If, however, athletes who feel a need for breaks continue training—instead of taking those breaks through appropriate multiactivity workouts—they risk injury and a real threat of losing ground in their training plans.

Athletes and advanced exercisers plan multiactivity workouts as a matter of habit, often not viewing the different activities in their workouts as separate but rather as naturally integrated, even though one or another usually predominates. Thus, a swim sprint or long-distance workout may be immediately preceded by a short walk, jog, or run and immediately followed by a complete and deliberate upper body stretching session, followed by an upper-body weight training session, and completed with an abdominal resistance workout. The entire workout may take 2 to 2-1/2 hours, but it's viewed as one multiactivity workout, because the elements are linked together to complement the *dominant theme* (in this instance, swimming).

Identifying the Dominant Theme

The *dominant theme* of a multiactivity workout is the single sport (e.g., swimming, running, cycling) or fitness element (cardiovascular, flexibility, muscular strength) you intend to enhance most by the combination of activities in the workout. In other words, the intention is to build the workout around the dominant theme.

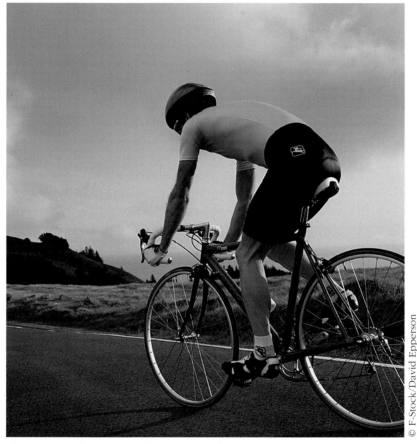

© F-Stock/David Epperson

Plan your workouts around a dominant theme.

Triathletes may need to make more than one activity of central importance when preparing for competition, but if you are constructing multiactivity workouts to begin to enhance and expand your training options, the rule of a single dominant theme is generally appropriate. Sometimes, the addition of deliberate stretching or flexibility work may be all you need to expand a single-focus workout to a multiactivity workout; sometimes the addition of "workout inventiveness" will suffice to enhance the overall goal of addressing the workout's dominant theme (see 'Constructing Multiactivity Workouts' in this chapter).

For all exercisers, multiactivity workouts must stress attention to proper form and technique but must also recognize the occasional need for levity to boost psychological and emotional commitment to training, as well as to provide a change of pace to exercising muscles. In order to help identify broad physical or emotional recovery needs, exercisers must listen to and accept the feedback from their exercising muscles and limbs.

Constructing Multiactivity Workouts

Depending on your orientation and dominant theme, you'll construct multiactivity workouts either to pump variety and fun into your workouts or to deliberately train your neuromuscular system and muscle-tendon-joint complexes to perform at a higher level of proficiency.

So get out pen and paper and be honest with yourself. Answer the following challenges and questions, making copious notes, because these will be highly instrumental when you are ready to set up multiactivity workouts to help meet your sport and fitness needs.

Identify why you want to use multiactivity workouts.   Are your race times disappointing? Are you getting injured too often? Are you overtraining one part of your body at the expense of another? Are you performing poorly in competition because you lack flexibility, stamina, strength, or cardiovascular endurance? Do you simply have a need for more variety and fun in your workouts?

Make a list of things you could do to add variety to your workout or activities to pursue that will help you meet your sport and fitness goals.   Don't hold anything back; for adding variety, list everything that's of interest to you, and for meeting fitness goals, be very specific about deficiencies in your training or sports/competitive performance.

Essentially, manipulating workouts means being clear about what you want to accomplish. If leg strength is your goal, there are numerous activities that will help you achieve this: running, walking, weight training, skipping, hopping, jumping rope, aerobics, hiking, cycling, stairclimbing, skating, nordic skiing, and even certain isometric type activities. Create lists like this for all you want to accomplish, and you'll have a broad menu of activities from which to choose.

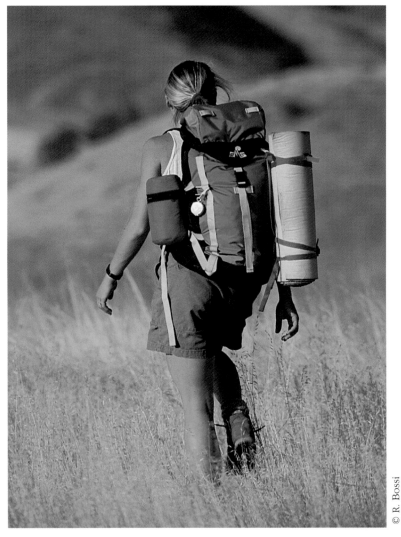

Add variety to your workouts by doing activities that complement your training plan.

Clearly, your power is in understanding how to manipulate workouts and to blend them in the correct proportions, even within the same exercise/activity discipline. There's no shortcut to learning this, and you can achieve it only through experience and experimentation. By following the general cross-training guidelines in this book, you should be able to blend activities in such a way that you enjoy and profit from the mix, including those ever-so-important, albeit infrequent, moments of training levity when laughter plays a leading role in the execution of activity.

Link activities that fit.   Once you've identified a list of activities that have some direct or indirect relation to your sport and fitness goals, try to link together the activities under your different sport and fitness goals. For example, under "stronger arms" you might list weight training, rowing, push-ups, tennis, handball, aerobics, chopping wood, and so forth. Some of these activities might also be listed under other goals, like "more agility" (under which handball, aerobics, and tennis could also be listed).

Other more general examples could be linking horseshoes with upper body work, swimming relays with interval training, terrain hiking with long-distance running, snowboarding with waterskiing, or surfing with either of the last two.

Make up three multiactivity workouts, and schedule them for the following week.   In designing the workouts, pay attention to the transitions between the activities and the need for equipment or other necessities. Multiactivity workouts may take all variety of shapes: a 45-minute walk, followed by a 10-minute stretch, followed by 3 hours of surfboarding, concluded with a brisk 15-minute ocean swim and brief upper body stretch. The dominant theme for such a workout could be overall fitness. This actual workout was one of my training workouts for the 2.4-mile Waikiki Roughwater Swim in Hawaii.

Multiactivity Workouts for a Multisport Athlete

Using the workouts in chapters 6 through 11 for reference, the following depicts a sample 5-day training schedule for a multisport athlete who competes on Sundays. Competition may be a triathlon, biathlon, community-specific race (such as canoeing and cycling, running and in-line skating, etc.), or any other multisport competition.

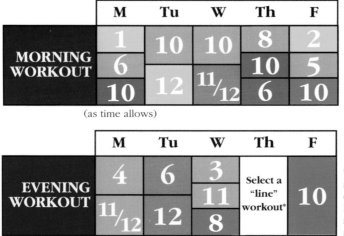

	M	Tu	W	Th	F
MORNING WORKOUT	1 6 10	10 12	10 11/12	8 10 6	2 5 10

(as time allows)

	M	Tu	W	Th	F
EVENING WORKOUT	4 11/12	6 12	3 11 8	Select a "line" workout*	10

*i.e., choose 2-6 activities of short duration at different levels of intensity and do them in succession

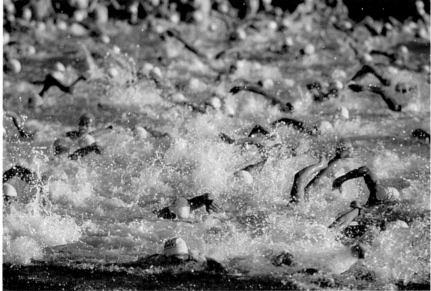

Competing in a triathlon is the goal for many cross-trainers.

Seven Key Training Concepts for Triathlon-Oriented Multisport Competitors

1. Your base work (fitness foundation) weekly totals should exceed the intended race distance by 3 to 4 times before you begin to hone your training for race day.

2. Again, with a sufficient fitness base, allow 2-1/2 to 3 months to prepare for any major multisport competition, like the triathlon. If you lack a sufficient base, allow 4 to 5 months to prepare for major competition.

3. Use a periodization model to build your base and to hone your technique and racing skills.

4. Work out at least twice a week in each discipline in the competition.

5. Use plenty of overdistance work to build endurance; long and slow works well in running, long and a consistent pushing pace works well in swimming, long and consistent spinning of the wheels works well in cycling.

6. Use hills, wind, rough water, pull buoys, and other forms of resistance to build and increase your natural competitive strength.

7. Train for the physical and mental transition between events. "Bricks" is a popular training technique where, for example, you might ride for 10 miles, hop off the bike and run 1 mile, and so forth in appropriate combinations. Thermal transitions in swimming may also be required when an open-water swim portion of a triathlon occurs in water substantially colder than your training water and no wet suit is worn. In such transitions, acclimation is important, but the focus must be on breathing consistency.

In the final chapter, you'll find an appropriate model for tracking your progress as a cross-trainer—tracking both how well you are doing and how good you are feeling!

14

Charting Your Progress

It's relatively easy for competitors to measure progress by simply comparing times and performances from race to race and from training session to training session. Nevertheless, every competitor realizes that a time for a 2-mile swim in *fast* water (smooth and buoyant) cannot be accurately compared to the same distance swim in a wind-blown lake or rough ocean; the same is true for a fast run or bike (no wind, or "flat hills").

Put simply, no course is the same on any given day (given no environmental controls). This being the case, competitors who want to chart their course and progress must develop a number of objective and subjective measures of evaluation. All levels of exercisers can profit from the same evaluative principles.

What Are Your Training Traits?

Because we don't all think the same way, we shouldn't attempt to chart our progress in exactly the same way. To focus more closely on how you might be inclined to view your cross-training progress, review your training traits in Table 14.1. By determining your slant toward right- or left-brain influence, you may gain additional insight on how to proportion the objective and subjective measures of evaluation we'll be reviewing in the next section.

Table 14.1	
Brain Hemispheres and Training Traits	
Left brain	*Right brain*
• Logical	• Creative
• Linear	• Spatial
• Narrowly defined goals	• Umbrella-shaped goals/ thoughts
• Stick to the training plan	
• Rest until you're healed when injured	• Complementary biomechanical development
• Training is work	• Versatile
• Working out and play don't mix	• Training is essential (so if injured, training is modified)
• Perfect one activity at a time	• Training needs to accommo- date changing life schedules
• Flexibility is a step-by-step process for one area of the body at a time	• Self-regulation is the discipline of training

The more right-brain inclined you are, the more you need to include subjective measures in the evaluation of your progress; the more left-brain inclined, the more you need to use objective measures. Each of these methods of evaluation may require modifications in your actual cross-training regimen and in the level of multiactivity workouts in your program.

The most important reason for some measure of evaluation of your progress is personal achievement. People measure this in a host of different ways, and I encourage you to carefully and honestly make those choices for yourself. For one person, achievement may be the act of completing a workout; for another, it may be only when he or she posts a personal best in a workout endeavor.

The following are a number of possible objective and subjective measures by which you may evaluate your progress with cross-training.

Objective Measures

The spectrum of objective measures may include

- performance times on measured, environmentally controlled courses;
- distances covered in set intervals of time;
- timed performances in controlled agility tests;
- flexibility measurements;
- assorted body measurements; and
- body weight as depicted on a scale. (Because body weight fluctuates constantly, weighing may not be a reliable evaluative measure, due to inherent inaccuracies in measuring the quality of change.)

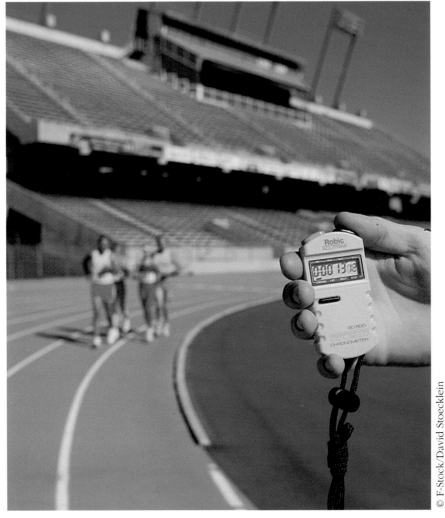

Elapsed time during a race or workout is one objective measure of performance.

Better ways to objectively measure body change include

- determining your body's percent body fat weight versus lean body weight,
- determining your achievement of the desired percentage of training heart rate during exercise,
- measuring your resting pulse and your recovery heart rate,
- gauging your level of strength—measured in the amount of weight you can lift in any particular exercise—and
- ascertaining your level of endurance in different activities.

Other objective measures may include

- competition awards (however, these may be misleading when you win an award with no challenging competition in your age group),
- any assortment of data collection on your activities, and
- meeting your planned training goals.

Finally, two methods of objectively assessing your performance and progress include

- analyzing your "race handicapping" and
- looking over your medical records.

Regarding handicapping, by comparing your times to those of a teammate's, training partner's, or a top finisher's, you may be able to gauge the relative merit of your performance, considering the race conditions as they apply to all competitors.

With respect to your medical records, the types, number, and timing of your injuries may reveal telltale trends. For example, a number of prerace injuries may be more psychosomatic than physical, or they may mean that you don't know how to or simply do not bother to taper your training before a race.

Subjective Measures

The spectrum of subjective measures may include

- your "feel" of the workout or competition,
- your level of anticipation for and your sense of achievement during the workout or competition,
- your assessment of the dynamics of a given activity and how it flowed (in other words, the way you felt about the transitions between activities or about the start or finish of a race), or
- your assessment of how focused or distracted you were while working out or competing.

Other subjective measures might involve

- the "look" of your body/contour/body part,
- the fit and feel of your clothing (especially those clothes that you know fit you best when you're in good shape),
- the "spring" (or lack of same) you feel in your walk or run,
- the look of your exercise posture in the eyes of others you admire or respect,
- your sense of coordination or agility,
- your level of confidence and changes in it with respect to workouts or competition, and
- your "ego comfort"—the level of comfort you have performing certain exercises or activities in front of others, whether they are strangers or friends.

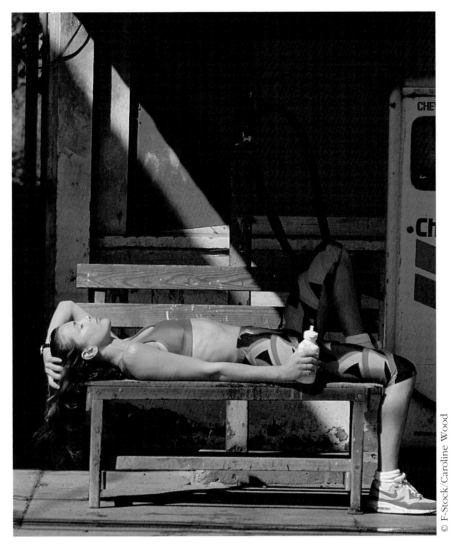

Simply assessing how you feel at the end of a workout is a good subjective measure of your training effectiveness.

Creating a Training Log

You have many options to choose from when deciding how precise you want to be in setting up a method for charting your progress. First, you must assess your right- or left-brain inclinations, then select your objective or subjective measures (probably everyone would profit from the inclusion of both kinds), and finally, bring your efforts into focus.

One way to focus your efforts is to establish a series of fitness goals that represent what you're trying to accomplish. Frame these goals in your language; make them suit your specific wants and needs. They're not cast in stone, so have fun with them. Once you've identified your goals, list the objective and subjective measures you'll use to chart your progress toward meeting them. Hopefully, the cross-training program you devised earlier was designed with these goals in mind.

A sample training log follows to provide you with an example of how to set up a tool with which to chart your cross-training progress. I've also included a blank format for you to make multiple copies of, so you can use them to create an easy-to-carry evaluation notebook in which to keep notes on your progress.

Training Log

Fitness goal: To increase my overall upper body strength and size by 20% in 6 months, as measured by my ability to lift heavier weights in seven lifts.

Objective measures	Current weight lifted	Weight lifted at 6 weeks	Weight lifted at 12 weeks	Weight lifted at 18 weeks	Weight lifted at 24 weeks
Bench press					
Incline press					
Military press					
Upright row					
Dumbbell fly					
Biceps curls					
Triceps press					

Subjective notes:

Workout date	Selected subjective observations
5/4/94	1. Feel awkward in gym when the heavy lifters are there. Need to change workout time.
7/12/94	2. Am feeling better about my form in the bench since I widened my grip.
8/30/94	3. Got a compliment today from Sally about my lats; she's a great role model—I'm pumped!

Another example, more abbreviated:

Fitness goal: To shape and tone my body, and reduce my percentage of body fat within 6 months.

Training Log					
Fitness goal:					
Objective measures	Current weight lifted	Weight lifted at 6 weeks	Weight lifted at 12 weeks	Weight lifted at 18 weeks	Weight lifted at 24 weeks

Subjective notes:

Workout date   **Selected subjective observations**

1.

2.

3.

Overall, the key to evaluating your progress is carefully identifying what you desire to accomplish (and feel a need to evaluate) and finding a way to do it. The examples in these training logs were ideally suited to that kind of evaluation. Some people, though, will want a day-to-day subjective assessment of certain elements of their overall fitness cross-training program, and if you are so inclined (and disinclined to taking measurements, etc.), you might find the Reflective Training Log more to your liking.

Reflective Training Log			
Date	**Planned activity**	**Actual Activity**	**Reflections**
_____	_____	_____	_____
_____	_____	_____	_____
_____	_____	_____	_____
_____	_____	_____	_____
_____	_____	_____	_____
_____	_____	_____	_____

In Conclusion

Why bother measuring aspects of your progress? The benefit comes in gaining feedback on how well your efforts are working to help you accomplish your fitness goals and how darn good (or frustrated) you feel about the activities and effort. Nonetheless, too much attention to achievement, given the often tough task of changing the effects of years of poor health and poor exercise habits in a relatively short time, is self-defeating.

Even worse than the risk of failure is the risk of losing sight of how good it feels to be doing something novel and active. How you feel about pitching a horseshoe, tugging on a rope in a spirited tug-of-war, running your first marathon, or taking your first alpine lake swim in 50-degree water is measurably more important in the big picture. Feel good about what you're doing, and why you're doing it, and the results will always be appreciated.

Index

A

Abdominal resistance work
  orange zone, 114
  red zone, 128
Abdominals, stretching exercises for, 42
Abdominal work, transition from
    stairclimbing, 32-33
Achilles tendon and posterior lower leg,
    stretching exercises for, 39
Aerobics
  aerobics class behind/in front of the
    instructor (purple zone), 84
  benefits of cross-training for, 7
  step aerobics (orange zone), 112
  step aerobics class (red zone), 126
  video aerobics (blue zone), 72
  video aerobics (green zone), 58, 62
  video aerobics with partner (orange
    zone), 111
  video aerobics with partner (yellow
    zone), 98
Ankles and lower leg, stretching exercises
    for, 38-39

B

Back, lower, stretching exercises for, 41
Back workouts, 113, 127
Beginning/easy exercisers benefiting from
    cross-training, 5
  characteristics of, 5
  one month cross-training program
    for, 136
Blue zone workouts, 63-74
  after injury, 63
  expert's uses of, 74
  specific instructions, 64-73
  summary table, 74
  using, 63
  for weight management, 63

Body composition, 10-12
  acceptable range of body fat, 10-12
  reducing body fat levels with cross
    training, 12
Body fat, 10-12
Borg scale, to determine RPE, 27
Brain hemispheres, and training traits,
    151-152
Buttocks and hips, stretching exercises
    for, 41

C

Caloric demands, estimated for different
    exercises, 47-48
Calorie management, 47-48
Cardiovascular fitness, exercising for, 8
Charting progress, 151-158
  objective measures, 152-154
  subjective measures, 154
Chest workouts
  chest blasts (orange zone), 113
  chest blasts (red zone), 127
  with free weights (purple zone), 86
  with free weights (yellow zone), 100
Clothing for cross-training, 15
Competitive/intense exercisers
  benefiting from cross-training, 5
  characteristics of, 5
  one month cross-training program
    for, 138
  specific workouts for competition, 138
Cross-training
  advantages of, 3
  assessing readiness for, 22-25
  beginning/easy exercisers benefiting
    from, 5
  benefits of, for different activities, 7
  charting personal progress, 151-158
  checking level of fitness before
    participation, 21-27

Cross-training *(continued)*
 competitive/intense exercisers benefiting
  from, 5
 fitness components of, 7-12
 frequent/moderate exercisers
  benefiting from, 5
 guidelines for varying climates and
  conditions, 18-20
 importance of manipulating mode,
  intensity, frequency and duration, 34
 importance of proper mechanics and
  form, 34
 measures of progress, 152-154
 mixing workouts effectively, 29-34
 multiple activity workouts, 143-150
 objective measures of progress, 152, 154
 preparation and planning essential to, 2
 preparticipation checklist, 22
 promoting flexibility, 36
 reducing risk of injury, 4-5
 rest important in, 3
 role of, 1-2
 subjective measures of progress, 154
 training log for, 155-158
 warming up and cooling down, 35-43
 warming up essential, 35-37
Cross-training apparel, 13-16
Cross-training equipment, costs of, 16-18
Cross-training programs
 advantages and disadvantages of training
  partners, 135
 for all-round fitness, 140
 APPEAL framework for, 133-135
 beginning/easy program, 136
 for competition, 140
 competitive/intense program, 138
 concepts for setting up a one-month
  program, 135-138
 frequent/moderate program, 137
 periodization applied to, 139
 planning a 12-month program, 139-141
 setting up a personal program, 133-141
Cross-training workouts,
 blue zone workouts, 63-74
 green zone workouts, 49-62
 manipulating intensity in, 75
 multiple activity workouts, 143-150
 orange zone workouts, 103-116
 purple zone workouts, 75-88
 red zone workouts, 117-130
 yellow zone workouts, 89-102
Cross-training workout zones, 45-48. *See
 also* Specific zones
 constructing a training program with,
  131-132
 defined by intensity and duration, 45-46
 making correct choices, 46-47
Cycling
 adapting to gear changes, 55

 benefits of cross-training for, 6
 distance ride (orange zone), 109
 distance ride (red zone), 124
 Fartlek ride (purple zone), 81
 Fartlek ride (yellow zone), 96
 hill-climb cycling (purple zone), 80
 hill-climb cycling (yellow zone), 95
 mile ride X 2 (green zone), 55
 mile ride X 4 (blue zone), 68
 stationary ride (blue zone), 69
 timed-interval ride (orange zone), 108
 timed-interval ride (red zone), 123
 transition to running, 32
D
Duration. *See also* Cross-training workout
  zones
 importance of manipulating, 34
 varieties of, in workout zones, 45-46
E
Exercise, caloric demands of, 47-48
Exercise goals, 5
Exercise intensity. *See* Intensity
Exercise transitions
 from cycling to running, 32
 flexibility easing, 36
 green zone workouts as, 49-50
 helping, 31-34
 and muscle specificity, 30-31
 from stairclimbing to abdominal work,
  32-33
 from swimming to upper body weight
  training, 32
 tips for, 32-33
Eyewear for cross-training, 15-16
F
Fitness components of cross-training, 7-12
 body composition, 10-12
 cardiovascular fitness, 8
 flexibility, 12
 muscular endurance, 10
 muscular strength, 8-10
Fitness level
 choosing appropriate workout zones, 46
 yellow zone workouts increasing, 89
Flexibility, 12
 easing transition, 36
 importance of stretching, 12
 improved by stretching, 38
 promoting, 36
Free weight, workouts using, 86, 100
Frequent/moderate exercisers
 benefiting from cross-training, 5
 characteristics of, 5
 one month cross-training program
  for, 137
G
Gloves for cross-training, 15
Green zone workouts, 49-62

converting to purple, 76
experts' uses for, 61
to introduce new activities, 50
specific instructions, 51-60
summary table, 62
as training holiday, 50
as transitions, 49-50
using, 49-50

H

Hamstrings, stretching exercises for, 40
Headgear for cross-training, 16
Heart rate
determining maximum heart rate, 25
and rating of perceived exertion, 26-27
resting, 8
RPE paralleling training heart rate
ranges, 27
taking pulse, 8, 25
target, 25-27

I

Injury
from failure to warm up, 35, 37
inadequate warming up inviting, 35
risk reduced by cross-training, 4-5
using blue zone workouts following, 63
Intensity. See also Cross-training workout
zones
importance of manipulating, 34, 75
levels of, in workout zones, 45-46
rating of perceived exertion to
measure, 26-27

K

Knees, back of, stretching exercises for, 40

L

Lateral shoulders, stretching exercises
for, 42
Lower back, stretching exercises for, 41

M

Maximum heart rate, determining, 25
Multiple activity workouts, 143-150
adding variety to, 146-147
advantages of, 143-145
constructing, 146-148
dominant theme for, 145-146
example of, 148
form, technique, and levity all important
to, 146
key training concepts for triathlon-
oriented multisport competitors,
149-150
linking activities, 148
reasons for using, 146
Muscles, creating program to maximize
range of motion, 31
Muscle specificity, and exercise transitions,
30-31
Muscular endurance, 10

cross-training preferred for
developing, 10
workouts developing, 59, 60
Muscular strength, 8-10
advantages of improving, 10

O

Orange zone workouts, 103-116
choosing familiar activities recom-
mended, 103-104
experts' uses of, 115
specific instructions, 105-114
summary table, 116
testing ability during, 104
using, 103-104

P

Perceived exertion. See Rating of perceived
exertion
Periodization, 139
Purple zone workouts, 75-88
experts' uses of, 87
flexibility of, 76
introduction to, 75-76
manipulating intensity in, 75
specific instructions, 77-86
summary table, 88
using, 76

R

Rating of perceived exertion (RPE), 26-27
Borg scale to determine, 27
paralleling training heart rate ranges, 27
Red zone workouts, 117-130
challenge and risks of, 117
experts' uses of, 129
preparation essential for, 118
specific instructions, 119-128
summary table, 130
using, 117-118
Resistance machines, workouts using, 59,
73, 86, 99, 113
Rest, importance of, in cross-training, 3
Resting heart rate (RHR), as measure of
cardiovascular fitness, 8
Running
benefits of cross-training for, 5-6
distance run (red zone), 120
easy run (green zone), 51
fun terrain run (green zone), 52
incline-decline run (yellow zone), 91
long terrain run (blue zone), 65
paced-track-interval sprints (red
zone), 119
paced track interval workouts (orange
zone), 105
stair run/step-ups (purple zone), 78
stair run/step-ups (yellow zone), 92
timed long easy run (blue zone), 64
transition from cycling, 32
up and downhill run (purple
zone), 77

S

Safety considerations
  guidelines for cross-training in varying
    climates and conditions, 18-20
  guidelines for equipment, 13-16
Shoes for cross-training, 13-15
Shoulders, lateral, stretching exercises
  for, 42
Shoulder workouts, 85, 99
Stairclimbing, transition to abdominal
  work, 32-33
Stretching
  essential for healthy cross-training, 37-38
  importance of, 12
  tips for, 37-38
Stretching exercises, 38-43
Swimming
  baby pyramid sprint swim X 2 (yellow
    zone), 94
  benefits of cross-training for, 7
  paced sprints (purple zone), 79
  paced sprints (yellow zone), 93
  pull, swim, kick (orange zone), 106
  pull, swim, kick (red zone), 121
  pyramid swim (orange zone), 107
  pyramid swim (red zone), 122
  swim doubles (green zone), 53
  swim doubles plus (blue zone), 66
  swim/pull buoy doubles plus (blue
    zone), 67
  swim/pull buoy doubles (green zone),
    54
  transition to upper body weight training,
    32

T

Target heart rate, 25-27
Training heart rate
  and orange zone workouts, 103-104
  paralleling RPE, 27
Training log, 155-158
Training traits, 151-154
Transitions. *See* Exercise transitions
Triathletes
  key training concepts for, 149-150
  specific muscle training needed by, 10
Triceps, stretching exercises for, 42-43

V

Video aerobics, 58, 72, 98, 111

W

Walking
  adventurous terrain walk (blue zone), 71
  benefits of cross-training for, 7
  distance walk (red zone), 125
  easy walk (green zone), 56
  fun terrain walk (green zone), 57
  hill-climb walking (purple zone), 82
  long easy walk (blue zone), 70
  paced track intervals (orange zone), 110
  stair climb/step-ups (purple zone), 83
  stair climb/step-ups (yellow zone), 97
Warming up
  approaches to, 35-36
  importance of, 35
  including stretching, 36
  slow pace essential, 36-37
  stretching tips, 37-38
  taking stock during, 36-37
Weather, guidelines for cross-training in
  varying climates and conditions, 18-20
Weight management, 10-12
  aided by cross-training, 12
  using blue zone workouts for, 63
  workouts aiding, 64, 70
Weight training
  benefits of cross-training for, 7
  caloric costs of, 47-48
  mixing effectively, 29-30
  planning transitional activities, 30-34
  purpose, participation, and practicality
    considerations, 47
  transition from swimming to upper body
    weight training, 32
  workouts using weights, 60, 73, 86, 100
Workout zones. *See* Cross-training workout
  zones

Y

Yellow zone workouts, 89-102
  best for improving basic fitness level, 89
  cardiovascular benefits from, 89
  experts' uses of, 101
  integrating into workout plan, 90
  not for new activities, 90
  specific instructions, 91-100
  summary table, 102
  using, 89-90

About
the Author

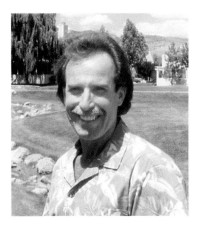

John Yacenda is an accomplished athlete and educator. He has coached and taught many sports since 1975, including football, soccer, baseball, track and field, skiing, swimming, and snowboarding.

Dr. Yacenda is the author of *High Performance Skiing* and *Alpine Skiing*, as well as more than 1,800 articles and columns on fitness-related topics. He has been a contributing editor for *Let's Live* magazine since 1984 and was a contributing editor for *Fitness Management* and *Natural Life* magazines for 5 years. He writes a weekly ski column that appears in newspapers in Colorado, Nevada, and California and throughout the Lake Tahoe area. In 1975, he earned his doctorate in health education and psychology from The Union Institute in Cincinnati. From 1971 to 1986, he taught health sciences at several California colleges and universities. Now he devotes more time to cross-training, competing in various sports, and writing about sports and cross-training. He is also the program manager of the HIV/AIDS Program Office for the Nevada State Health Division.

Yacenda cross-trains and competes throughout the year, and in the summer he enjoys international and United States Masters Swimming sanctioned open- and rough-water competitions. The Family YMCA and the Sports West Athletic Club in Reno are his two homes-away-from-home.

...ss books from Human Kinetics

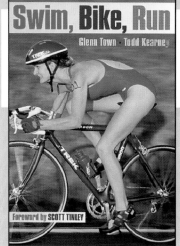

Glenn Town and Todd Kearney

Foreword by Scott Tinley

1994 • Paper • 240 pp
Item PTOW0513 • ISBN 0-87322-513-9
$15.95 ($21.50 Canadian)

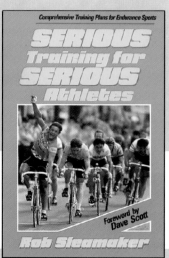

Rob Sleamaker

*Foreword by Dave Scott,
6-time winner of the Ironman Triathlon*

1989 • Paper • 264 pp
Item PSLE0338 • ISBN 0-88011-338-3
$15.95 ($21.50 Canadian)

Thomas R. Baechle, EdD, CSCS, and Barney R. Groves, PhD, CSCS

1992 • Paper • 208 pp • Item PBAE0451
ISBN 0-88011-451-7 • $14.95 ($19.95 Canadian)

Plus these titles* in the Fitness Spectrum Series:

- Fitness Aerobics
- Fitness Aquatics
- Fitness Cycling
- Fitness Running
- Fitness Walking
- Fitness Weight Training

*Some of these books are forthcoming.
Call for availability dates.

Place your order using the appropriate telephone number/address
shown on page iv of this book,
or **call toll-free in the U.S. (1-800-747-4457).**

Human Kinetics
The Information Leader in Physical Activity

2335

Prices are subject to change.